Introduction

Welcome to ***"100 Vegetarian Recipes for Soothing Diverticulitis Symptoms."*** This cookbook is a comprehensive guide designed to support individuals navigating the challenges of diverticulitis while adhering to a vegetarian diet.

Diverticulitis, a condition characterized by inflamed pouches in the colon, can be uncomfortable and disruptive to daily life. Managing this condition often involves dietary adjustments to alleviate symptoms and promote digestive health. While traditional approaches may emphasize bland, low-fiber diets, this cookbook offers a fresh perspective by showcasing the diverse and flavorful world of vegetarian cuisine.

Our goal is to empower you to take control of your health and well-being through delicious, plant-based meals. Whether you're newly diagnosed or seeking new culinary inspiration on your journey with diverticulitis, this book is here to guide you. Each recipe has been carefully crafted with your needs in mind, focusing on ingredients that are gentle on the digestive system while providing essential nutrients and satisfying flavors.

In addition to the recipes, you'll find practical tips and guidance for managing diverticulitis through diet. We'll explore the importance of fiber, hydration, and gut-friendly ingredients, helping you make informed choices that support your digestive health.

With 100 vegetarian recipes ranging from comforting soups and stews to vibrant salads and nourishing grain bowls, there's something for every palate and occasion. Whether you're craving a hearty meal to soothe symptoms during a flare-up or seeking light and refreshing options for everyday wellness, you'll find inspiration within these pages.

We believe that food should not only nourish the body but also delight the senses and bring joy to the table. By embracing the abundance of vegetarian ingredients available to us, we can create meals that promote healing, vitality, and overall well-being.

Thank you for embarking on this culinary journey with us. Here's to delicious food, vibrant health, and thriving with diverticulitis.

1. Vegetable soup

Ingredients:
- 2 tablespoons olive oil
- 1 onion, diced
- 2 cloves garlic, minced
- 2 carrots, diced
- 2 celery stalks, diced
- 1 bell pepper, diced
- 1 zucchini, diced
- 1 cup diced tomatoes (fresh or canned)
- 4 cups vegetable broth
- 1 teaspoon dried thyme
- 1 teaspoon dried oregano
- Salt and pepper to taste
- Optional: 1 cup cooked beans (such as kidney beans or chickpeas)
- Optional: Fresh parsley or basil for garnish

Instructions:

1. Heat the olive oil in a large pot over medium heat. Add the onion and garlic and sauté until fragrant, about 2-3 minutes.

2. Add the carrots, celery, bell pepper, and zucchini to the pot. Cook, stirring occasionally, for about 5 minutes until the vegetables begin to soften.

3. Stir in the diced tomatoes, vegetable broth, dried thyme, and dried oregano. Bring the soup to a simmer.

4. Reduce the heat to low and let the soup simmer for about 20-25 minutes, or until the vegetables are tender.

5. If using, add the cooked beans to the soup and let them heat through, about 5 minutes.

6. Season the soup with salt and pepper to taste.

7. Ladle the soup into bowls and garnish with fresh parsley or basil if desired. Serve hot and enjoy!

Feel free to customize this recipe by adding other vegetables you have on hand or adjusting the seasoning to your taste preferences. Enjoy your homemade vegetable soup!

2. Lentil soup

Ingredients:
- 2 tablespoons olive oil
- 1 onion, diced
- 2 cloves garlic, minced
- 2 carrots, diced
- 2 celery stalks, diced
- 1 cup dried lentils (green or brown), rinsed
- 1 can (14.5 oz) diced tomatoes, with juice
- 4 cups vegetable broth
- 2 cups water
- 1 teaspoon ground cumin
- 1 teaspoon ground coriander
- 1/2 teaspoon smoked paprika
- 1/2 teaspoon dried thyme
- 1 bay leaf
- Salt and pepper to taste
- Optional: 1 cup chopped spinach or kale
- Optional: Fresh lemon juice and chopped parsley for garnish

Instructions:
1. Heat the olive oil in a large pot over medium heat. Add the diced onion and cook until softened, about 5 minutes.

2. Add the minced garlic, carrots, and celery to the pot. Cook, stirring occasionally, until the vegetables begin to soften, about 5-7 minutes.

3. Stir in the lentils, diced tomatoes (with juice), vegetable broth, water, ground cumin, ground coriander, smoked paprika, dried thyme, and bay leaf.

4. Bring the soup to a boil, then reduce the heat to low. Cover and let it simmer for about 30-40 minutes, or until the lentils are tender.

5. If using, add the chopped spinach or kale to the pot and let it wilt, about 5 minutes.

6. Remove the bay leaf and season the soup with salt and pepper to taste.

7. If desired, add a squeeze of fresh lemon juice to brighten the flavors. Garnish with chopped parsley. Ladle the soup into bowls and serve hot. Enjoy!

This lentil soup is perfect for a cozy meal and can be easily customized with your favorite vegetables and spices. Enjoy!

3. Miso soup with tofu

Ingredients:
- 4 cups water
- 4 tablespoons miso paste (white or red, depending on your preference)
- 1 block (about 14 oz) firm tofu, cubed
- 2 green onions, thinly sliced
- 1 sheet nori (seaweed), cut into thin strips (optional)
- 1 cup sliced mushrooms (shiitake, button, or your choice)
- 1 tablespoon soy sauce or tamari
- 1 teaspoon sesame oil (optional)
- Optional additions: cooked soba noodles, spinach, bok choy, or other vegetables of your choice

Instructions:
1. In a pot, bring the water to a gentle simmer over medium heat.

2. While the water is heating, prepare the tofu by cutting it into small cubes and slicing the green onions.

3. Once the water is simmering, add the sliced mushrooms to the pot and let them cook for a few minutes until they begin to soften.

4. In a small bowl, whisk together the miso paste with a ladleful of the hot water until the miso is dissolved and smooth.

5. Add the dissolved miso paste to the pot and stir well to combine. Let the soup simmer gently for a few more minutes.

6. Add the cubed tofu to the pot and let it heat through for about 2-3 minutes.

7. Stir in the soy sauce or tamari for seasoning. If using, add the sesame oil for extra flavor.

8. Taste the soup and adjust the seasoning if needed.

9. Just before serving, add the sliced green onions and nori strips to the pot. Give the soup a final stir. Ladle the miso soup into bowls and serve hot. Enjoy!

Feel free to customize this soup by adding your favorite vegetables or adjusting the seasoning according to your taste preferences. It's a versatile and nourishing dish that's perfect for any occasion!

4. Quinoa salad with roasted vegetables

Ingredients:
- 1 cup quinoa, rinsed
- 2 cups water or vegetable broth
- 2 tablespoons olive oil
- 2 cloves garlic, minced
- 1 teaspoon dried herbs
(such as thyme, rosemary, or oregano)
- Salt and pepper to taste
- 2 tablespoons balsamic vinegar
- 2 cups mixed vegetables (such as bell peppers, zucchini, cherry tomatoes, red onion, etc.), chopped into bite-sized pieces
- 1/4 cup chopped fresh herbs (such as parsley, basil, or cilantro)
- Juice of 1 lemon
- Optional: crumbled feta cheese or goat cheese
- Optional: toasted nuts or seeds (such as almonds, walnuts, or sunflower seeds)

Instructions:
1. Preheat your oven to 400°F (200°C).

2. In a saucepan, combine the quinoa and water or vegetable broth. Bring to a boil, then reduce the heat to low, cover, and simmer for about 15-20 minutes, or until the quinoa is cooked and the liquid is absorbed. Remove from heat and let it sit, covered, for 5 minutes. Fluff the quinoa with a fork and transfer it to a large salad bowl to cool.

3. While the quinoa is cooking, prepare the roasted vegetables. Place the chopped vegetables on a baking sheet lined with parchment paper. Drizzle with olive oil, minced garlic, dried herbs, salt, and pepper. Toss to coat evenly.

4. Roast the vegetables in the preheated oven for about 20-25 minutes, or until they are tender and lightly browned, stirring halfway through cooking.

5. Once the quinoa has cooled slightly and the roasted vegetables are done, add the vegetables to the bowl with the quinoa.

6. In a small bowl, whisk together the lemon juice, balsamic vinegar, and chopped fresh herbs to make the dressing. Pour the dressing over the quinoa and roasted vegetables, and toss gently to combine.

7. If using, sprinkle the crumbled feta cheese or goat cheese over the salad, along with toasted nuts or seeds for added crunch.

8. Serve the quinoa salad immediately, or refrigerate it for a few hours to allow the flavors to meld. Enjoy!

This quinoa salad with roasted vegetables is perfect for a light lunch or dinner, and it's also great for meal prep. Feel free to customize it with your favorite vegetables and toppings!

5. Greek salad with feta cheese

Ingredients:
- 4 large tomatoes, chopped
- 1 cucumber, peeled and sliced
- 1 green bell pepper, sliced
- 1 red onion, thinly sliced
- 1/2 cup Kalamata olives
- 200g (about 7 oz) feta cheese, cut into large cubes or crumbled
- 1 teaspoon dried oregano
- Salt and pepper to taste
- 1/4 cup extra virgin olive oil
- 1-2 tablespoons red wine vinegar
- Optional: fresh oregano or parsley for garnish

Instructions:
1. In a large salad bowl, combine the chopped tomatoes, cucumber slices, sliced green bell pepper, and thinly sliced red onion.

2. Add the Kalamata olives to the bowl.

3. Gently toss the vegetables and olives together.

4. Place the feta cheese on top of the salad. You can either cut the feta into large cubes or crumble it, depending on your preference.

5. Sprinkle the dried oregano over the salad, and season with salt and pepper to taste. Be cautious with the salt, as the feta cheese and olives are already salty.

6. Drizzle the extra virgin olive oil and red wine vinegar over the salad.

7. Toss the salad gently to combine all the ingredients and coat them with the dressing.

8. If desired, garnish with fresh oregano or parsley.

9. Serve immediately and enjoy!

This Greek salad is a perfect accompaniment to grilled meats or fish, or it can be enjoyed on its own as a light and healthy meal.

6. Spinach and feta quiche

Ingredients:
- 2 cups fresh spinach, roughly chopped
- 1 cup crumbled feta cheese
- 1/2 cup shredded mozzarella cheese (optional)
- 1/4 cup grated Parmesan cheese
- 1 tablespoon olive oil
- 1 small onion, finely chopped
- 2 cloves garlic, minced

- 1 pre-made pie crust (9-inch), thawed if frozen
- 6 large eggs
- 1 cup milk (whole milk or any milk of your choice)
- 1/2 cup heavy cream (or substitute with more milk)
- 1/2 teaspoon salt
- 1/4 teaspoon black pepper
- 1/4 teaspoon nutmeg

Instructions:

1. Preheat your oven to 375°F (190°C).

2. Roll out the pie crust and carefully place it into a 9-inch pie dish. Press the crust into the bottom and up the sides of the dish. Trim any excess dough and crimp the edges if desired. Prick the bottom of the crust with a fork to prevent air bubbles from forming.

3. In a skillet, heat the olive oil over medium heat. Add the chopped onion and minced garlic, and sauté until softened and fragrant, about 3-4 minutes.

4. Add the chopped spinach to the skillet and cook until wilted, about 2-3 minutes. Remove from heat and let it cool slightly.

5. In a mixing bowl, whisk together the eggs, milk, heavy cream, salt, pepper, and nutmeg until well combined.

6. Spread the cooked spinach mixture evenly over the bottom of the pie crust.

7. Sprinkle the crumbled feta cheese over the spinach mixture, followed by the shredded mozzarella cheese if using.

8. Carefully pour the egg mixture over the spinach and cheese in the pie crust.

9. Sprinkle the grated Parmesan cheese evenly over the top of the quiche.

10. Place the quiche on a baking sheet to catch any potential spills, then transfer it to the preheated oven.

11. Bake the quiche for 35-40 minutes, or until the center is set and the top is golden brown. Remove the quiche from the oven and let it cool for a few minutes before slicing. Serve the spinach and feta quiche warm or at room temperature. Enjoy!

7. Baked sweet potatoes

Ingredients:
- 4 medium sweet potatoes
- Olive oil
- Salt
- Optional toppings: butter, cinnamon, brown sugar, maple syrup, chopped nuts, Greek yogurt, black beans, avocado, etc.

Instructions:
1. Preheat your oven to 400°F (200°C).

2. Scrub the sweet potatoes under running water to remove any dirt. Pat them dry with a clean kitchen towel.

3. Pierce each sweet potato several times with a fork or knife. This allows steam to escape while they bake and prevents them from bursting.

4. Rub each sweet potato with a small amount of olive oil. This helps to crisp up the skin and adds flavor.

5. Sprinkle each sweet potato with a pinch of salt.

6. Place the sweet potatoes on a baking sheet lined with parchment paper or aluminum foil, leaving space between them.

7. Bake the sweet potatoes in the preheated oven for 45-60 minutes, or until they are tender and easily pierced with a fork. The baking time will depend on the size and thickness of your sweet potatoes.

8. Once the sweet potatoes are baked, remove them from the oven and let them cool for a few minutes before serving.

9. To serve, slice each sweet potato lengthwise and fluff the flesh with a fork. Add your desired toppings such as butter, cinnamon, brown sugar, maple syrup, chopped nuts, Greek yogurt, black beans, avocado, etc.

10. Serve the baked sweet potatoes hot and enjoy!

Baked sweet potatoes are versatile and can be served as a side dish or as a main course with a variety of toppings. They're nutritious, delicious, and easy to make!

8. Grilled portobello mushrooms

Ingredients:
- 4 large portobello mushrooms
- 2-3 tablespoons balsamic vinegar
- 2-3 tablespoons olive oil
- 2 cloves garlic, minced
- 1 teaspoon dried thyme (or other herbs of your choice)
- Salt and pepper to taste
- Optional toppings: crumbled goat cheese, chopped fresh parsley, sliced tomatoes, balsamic glaze, etc.

Instructions:

1. Clean the portobello mushrooms by gently wiping them with a damp paper towel to remove any dirt. Avoid soaking them in water, as mushrooms can absorb excess moisture.

2. Remove the stems from the mushrooms and discard them, or save them for another use.

3. In a shallow dish or a large resealable plastic bag, whisk together the balsamic vinegar, olive oil, minced garlic, dried thyme, salt, and pepper to create a marinade.

4. Place the cleaned mushrooms in the marinade, making sure they are well coated. Allow them to marinate for at least 20-30 minutes, flipping them occasionally to ensure even coating.

5. Preheat your grill to medium-high heat.

6. Once the mushrooms have finished marinating, remove them from the marinade and shake off any excess.

7. Place the mushrooms on the preheated grill, gill-side down. Cook for 4-5 minutes on each side, or until they are tender and grill marks appear.

8. While grilling, you can brush the mushrooms with any remaining marinade for added flavor.

9. Once the mushrooms are cooked to your desired level of doneness, remove them from the grill and transfer them to a serving platter.

10. If desired, top the grilled portobello mushrooms with crumbled goat cheese, chopped fresh parsley, sliced tomatoes, balsamic glaze, or any other toppings of your choice. Serve the grilled portobello mushrooms immediately while hot. Enjoy!

Grilled portobello mushrooms are versatile and can be served as a side dish, on top of salads, in sandwiches, or even as a meat substitute in vegetarian dishes. They're delicious, easy to make, and perfect for outdoor grilling or indoor cooking.

9. Stuffed bell peppers with rice and beans

Ingredients:
- 4 large bell peppers (any color),
tops removed and seeds removed
- 1 cup cooked rice (white or brown)
- 1 cup cooked black beans
(or kidney beans, chickpeas, etc.)
- 1 cup corn kernels (fresh, canned, or frozen)
- 1 small onion, finely chopped
- 2 cloves garlic, minced
- 1 teaspoon ground cumin
- 1 teaspoon smoked paprika
- 1/2 teaspoon chili powder (adjust to taste)
- Salt and pepper to taste
- 1 cup shredded cheese (such as cheddar, Monterey Jack, or a Mexican cheese blend)
- Optional toppings: chopped fresh cilantro, avocado slices, sour cream, salsa, etc.

Instructions:
1. Preheat your oven to 375°F (190°C).

2. In a large skillet, heat some olive oil over medium heat. Add the chopped onion and minced garlic, and sauté until softened and fragrant, about 3-4 minutes.

3. Add the cooked rice, black beans, corn kernels, ground cumin, smoked paprika, chili powder, salt, and pepper to the skillet. Stir well to combine and cook for another 2-3 minutes to allow the flavors to meld. Remove from heat.

4. Place the hollowed-out bell peppers upright in a baking dish that's just large enough to hold them snugly.

5. Spoon the rice and bean mixture into each bell pepper until they are filled to the top.

6. Sprinkle shredded cheese over the top of each stuffed bell pepper.

7. Cover the baking dish with aluminum foil and bake in the preheated oven for 25-30 minutes, or until the bell peppers are tender and the cheese is melted and bubbly.

8. Remove the foil and bake for an additional 5-10 minutes to lightly brown the cheese, if desired.

9. Once the stuffed bell peppers are cooked through and the cheese is melted, remove them from the oven and let them cool for a few minutes.

10. Serve the stuffed bell peppers hot, garnished with optional toppings such as chopped fresh cilantro, avocado slices, sour cream, salsa, etc. Enjoy your delicious and nutritious stuffed bell peppers with rice and beans!

10. Eggplant Parmesan

Ingredients:
- 2 large eggplants, sliced
- Salt
- 2 cups breadcrumbs
- 1 cup grated Parmesan cheese
- 2 tsp dried Italian seasoning
- 4 large eggs, beaten
- Olive oil
- 3 cups marinara sauce
- 2 cups shredded mozzarella cheese
- Fresh basil leaves for garnish (optional)

Instructions:
1. Preheat oven to 375°F (190°C).

2. Salt eggplant slices, let sit, then pat dry.

3. Dip slices in beaten eggs, then coat in breadcrumb mixture.

4. Fry eggplant slices until golden brown, then drain.

5. Layer marinara sauce, eggplant, and mozzarella cheese in a baking dish.

6. Repeat layers, ending with cheese.

7. Bake covered for 25-30 mins, then uncovered for 5-10 mins until bubbly.

8. Garnish with fresh basil leaves before serving. Enjoy!

11. Zucchini noodles with marinara sauce

Ingredients:
- 4 medium zucchinis
- 2 cups marinara sauce (homemade or store-bought)
- 2 cloves garlic, minced
- 2 tablespoons olive oil
- Salt and pepper to taste
- Grated Parmesan cheese for garnish (optional)
- Fresh basil leaves for garnish (optional)

Instructions:
1. Using a spiralizer or a vegetable peeler, create zucchini noodles (zoodles) from the zucchinis. Set aside.

2. In a large skillet, heat olive oil over medium heat. Add minced garlic and cook until fragrant, about 1 minute.

3. Add the zucchini noodles to the skillet and sauté for 2-3 minutes, or until they are just tender but still crisp. Be careful not to overcook them.

4. Pour the marinara sauce over the zucchini noodles and toss until the noodles are evenly coated with the sauce. Cook for an additional 1-2 minutes to heat the sauce.

5. Season with salt and pepper to taste.

6. Remove the skillet from heat and transfer the zucchini noodles with marinara sauce to serving plates.

7. Garnish with grated Parmesan cheese and fresh basil leaves, if desired.

8. Serve hot and enjoy your delicious and nutritious zucchini noodles with marinara sauce!

This dish is low-carb, gluten-free, and packed with flavor. It's a great way to enjoy a lighter version of pasta with all the deliciousness of marinara sauce. Feel free to customize it by adding your favorite toppings or protein such as grilled chicken or shrimp.

12. Roasted cauliflower steaks

Ingredients:
- 1 large head of cauliflower
- Olive oil
- Salt and pepper to taste
- Optional seasonings: garlic powder, paprika, cumin, thyme, etc.
- Optional toppings: grated Parmesan cheese, chopped parsley, lemon zest, etc.

Instructions:
1. Preheat your oven to 400°F (200°C).

2. Remove the outer leaves from the cauliflower and trim the stem end, leaving the core intact.

3. Place the cauliflower head stem side down on a cutting board. Carefully slice it into 1-inch thick "steaks" from the top (stem) down through the core. You should be able to get 2-3 steaks from one head of cauliflower, depending on its size. Reserve any florets that fall off for another use.

4. Arrange the cauliflower steaks in a single layer on a baking sheet lined with parchment paper or aluminum foil.

5. Drizzle olive oil over the cauliflower steaks and use your hands or a brush to coat them evenly. Season with salt, pepper, and any optional seasonings of your choice.

6. Roast the cauliflower steaks in the preheated oven for 20-25 minutes, flipping halfway through cooking, until they are golden brown and tender.

7. If desired, sprinkle grated Parmesan cheese over the cauliflower steaks during the last few minutes of cooking for extra flavor.

8. Remove the roasted cauliflower steaks from the oven and transfer them to serving plates.

9. Garnish with chopped parsley, lemon zest, or any other toppings of your choice.

10. Serve hot and enjoy your delicious and nutritious roasted cauliflower steaks!

These cauliflower steaks make a fantastic vegetarian main course or side dish. They're versatile and can be customized with various seasonings and toppings to suit your taste preferences.

13. Stuffed acorn squash with quinoa and vegetables

Ingredients:
- 2 acorn squash, halved and seeds removed
- 1 cup quinoa
- 2 cups vegetable broth or water
- 1 tbsp olive oil
- 1 small onion, diced
- 2 cloves garlic, minced
- Assorted diced vegetables (carrot, celery, bell pepper)
- 1 cup chopped kale or spinach
- 1 tsp each dried thyme and sage
- Salt and pepper to taste
- Optional: chopped nuts, fresh parsley or cilantro for garnish

Instructions:
1. Preheat oven to 400°F (200°C). Roast acorn squash halves cut side down on a baking sheet for 25-30 minutes.

2. Cook quinoa in vegetable broth according to package instructions.

3. Sauté onion, garlic, and assorted vegetables in olive oil until tender.

4. Add kale/spinach, dried herbs, salt, and pepper. Cook until greens are wilted.

5. Stir cooked quinoa into the vegetable mixture. Optional: add chopped nuts.

6. Fill roasted squash halves with quinoa and vegetable mixture.

7. Bake filled squash halves for 10-15 minutes.

8. Garnish with fresh parsley or cilantro if desired.

9. Serve hot. Enjoy!

This condensed version still maintains all the essential steps and flavors of the dish.

14. Vegetable stir-fry with tofu

Ingredients:
- 14 oz (400g) firm tofu, drained and cubed
- 2 tablespoons soy sauce or tamari
- 2 tablespoons cornstarch
- 2 tablespoons vegetable oil
- 2 cloves garlic, minced
- 1 tablespoon grated ginger
- 4 cups mixed vegetables (such as bell peppers, broccoli, carrots, snap peas, mushrooms, etc.), sliced or chopped
- 1/4 cup vegetable broth or water
- 2 tablespoons oyster sauce or hoisin sauce (for vegetarian/vegan option)
- Cooked rice or noodles for serving
- Optional garnishes: sesame seeds, sliced green onions, cilantro

Instructions:
1. In a bowl, toss the tofu cubes with soy sauce (or tamari) until evenly coated. Sprinkle cornstarch over the tofu and toss again until coated.

2. Heat 1 tablespoon of vegetable oil in a large skillet or wok over medium-high heat. Add the tofu cubes and cook until golden brown and crispy on all sides, about 5-7 minutes. Remove tofu from the skillet and set aside.

3. In the same skillet, heat the remaining tablespoon of vegetable oil. Add minced garlic and grated ginger, and cook for about 1 minute until fragrant.

4. Add the mixed vegetables to the skillet and stir-fry for 5-7 minutes, or until they are crisp-tender.

5. Pour vegetable broth (or water) into the skillet to deglaze, scraping up any browned bits from the bottom.

6. Return the cooked tofu to the skillet and stir in oyster sauce (or hoisin sauce), tossing everything together until heated through.

7. Serve the vegetable stir-fry with tofu over cooked rice or noodles. Garnish with sesame seeds, sliced green onions, and cilantro if desired. Enjoy your delicious and nutritious vegetable stir-fry with tofu!

This stir-fry is versatile, so feel free to customize it with your favorite vegetables and sauces. It's a great way to enjoy a flavorful and satisfying meal packed with protein and veggies!

15. Chickpea curry

Ingredients:
- 2 tablespoons vegetable oil
- 1 onion, finely chopped
- 3 cloves garlic, minced
- 1 tablespoon grated ginger
- 2 teaspoons curry powder
- 1 teaspoon ground cumin
- 1 teaspoon ground coriander
- 1/2 teaspoon turmeric powder
- 1/4 teaspoon cayenne pepper (adjust to taste)
- 1 can (14 oz / 400g) diced tomatoes
- 1 can (14 oz / 400g) coconut milk
- 2 cans (14 oz / 400g each) chickpeas, drained and rinsed
- Salt and pepper to taste
- Fresh cilantro for garnish (optional)
- Cooked rice or naan bread for serving

Instructions:
1. Heat vegetable oil in a large skillet or pot over medium heat. Add chopped onion and cook until softened, about 5 minutes.

2. Add minced garlic and grated ginger to the skillet and cook for another 2 minutes until fragrant.

3. Stir in curry powder, ground cumin, ground coriander, turmeric powder, and cayenne pepper. Cook for 1 minute to toast the spices.

4. Pour in diced tomatoes with their juices and coconut milk. Stir to combine.

5. Add drained and rinsed chickpeas to the skillet. Stir well, then bring the mixture to a simmer.

6. Reduce the heat to low and let the curry simmer uncovered for about 15-20 minutes, stirring occasionally, until the sauce thickens slightly and the flavors meld together.

7. Taste and adjust seasoning with salt and pepper as needed. Serve the chickpea curry hot over cooked rice or with naan bread.

8. Garnish with fresh cilantro if desired. Enjoy your delicious and comforting chickpea curry!

16. Lentil stew

Ingredients:
- 1 tablespoon olive oil
- 1 onion, diced
- 2 carrots, diced
- 2 celery stalks, diced
- 3 cloves garlic, minced
- 1 cup dried lentils (green or brown), rinsed and drained
- 4 cups vegetable broth or water
- 1 can (14 oz / 400g) diced tomatoes
- 1 teaspoon dried thyme
- 1 teaspoon dried oregano
- 1 bay leaf
- Salt and pepper to taste
- Fresh parsley for garnish (optional)

Instructions:
1. Heat olive oil in a large pot over medium heat. Add diced onion, carrots, and celery. Cook until softened, about 5-7 minutes.

2. Add minced garlic to the pot and cook for another minute until fragrant.

3. Stir in dried lentils, vegetable broth (or water), diced tomatoes (with their juices), dried thyme, dried oregano, and bay leaf. Season with salt and pepper to taste.

4. Bring the mixture to a boil, then reduce the heat to low. Cover and simmer for about 20-25 minutes, or until the lentils are tender.

5. Once the lentils are cooked, taste and adjust seasoning if necessary. Remove the bay leaf from the pot.

6. If you prefer a thicker stew, you can use a potato masher or immersion blender to partially blend some of the lentils and vegetables.

7. Serve the lentil stew hot, garnished with fresh parsley if desired.

8. Enjoy your delicious and nutritious lentil stew!

This lentil stew is comforting, satisfying, and packed with protein and fiber. It's perfect for a cozy dinner on a chilly evening, and leftovers taste even better the next day!

17. Black bean soup

Ingredients:
- 2 tablespoons olive oil
- 1 onion, diced
- 2 carrots, diced
- 2 celery stalks, diced
- 3 cloves garlic, minced
- 2 cans (14 oz / 400g each) black beans, drained and rinsed
- 4 cups vegetable broth
- 1 can (14 oz / 400g) diced tomatoes
- 1 teaspoon ground cumin
- 1 teaspoon chili powder
- 1/2 teaspoon smoked paprika
- Salt and pepper to taste
- Juice of 1 lime
- Fresh cilantro for garnish (optional)
- Sour cream or Greek yogurt for garnish (optional)
- Sliced avocado for garnish (optional)
- Tortilla chips for serving (optional)

Instructions:

1. Heat olive oil in a large pot over medium heat. Add diced onion, carrots, and celery. Cook until softened, about 5-7 minutes.

2. Add minced garlic to the pot and cook for another minute until fragrant.

3. Stir in drained and rinsed black beans, vegetable broth, diced tomatoes (with their juices), ground cumin, chili powder, and smoked paprika. Season with salt and pepper to taste.

4. Bring the mixture to a boil, then reduce the heat to low. Cover and simmer for about 20-25 minutes, stirring occasionally.

5. Once the vegetables are tender and the flavors have melded together, use an immersion blender or transfer a portion of the soup to a blender and blend until smooth. (You can also skip this step if you prefer a chunkier soup.)

6. Stir in the lime juice just before serving.

7. Ladle the black bean soup into bowls and garnish with fresh cilantro, a dollop of sour cream or Greek yogurt, sliced avocado, and tortilla chips if desired. Serve hot and enjoy your delicious and satisfying black bean soup!

This black bean soup is comforting, nutritious, and perfect for a cozy meal. It's also great for meal prep and freezes well for future enjoyment!

18. Ratatouille

Ingredients:
- 2 tablespoons olive oil
- 1 onion, diced
- 2 cloves garlic, minced
- 1 eggplant, diced
- 2 zucchini, diced
- 1 yellow bell pepper, diced
- 1 red bell pepper, diced
- 2 tomatoes, diced
- 1 can (14 oz / 400g) diced tomatoes
- 1 teaspoon dried thyme
- 1 teaspoon dried oregano
- Salt and pepper to taste
- Fresh basil leaves for garnish (optional)

Instructions:
1. Heat olive oil in a large skillet or pot over medium heat. Add diced onion and cook until softened, about 5 minutes.

2. Add minced garlic to the skillet and cook for another minute until fragrant.

3. Add diced eggplant to the skillet and cook for 5-7 minutes, until softened.

4. Stir in diced zucchini, yellow bell pepper, and red bell pepper. Cook for another 5 minutes, until the vegetables are slightly tender.

5. Add diced fresh tomatoes, canned diced tomatoes (with their juices), dried thyme, and dried oregano to the skillet. Season with salt and pepper to taste.

6. Reduce the heat to low, cover, and simmer for about 20-25 minutes, stirring occasionally, until all the vegetables are tender and the flavors have melded together.

7. Taste and adjust seasoning if necessary.

8. Serve the ratatouille hot, garnished with fresh basil leaves if desired. Enjoy your delicious and colorful ratatouille!

This ratatouille is a versatile dish that can be served as a side dish, over cooked grains like rice or quinoa, or even as a topping for pasta. It's a celebration of fresh summer vegetables and makes for a satisfying and nutritious meal.

19. Caprese salad with fresh mozzarella

Ingredients:
- 2 large ripe tomatoes, sliced
- 1 ball fresh mozzarella cheese, sliced
- Fresh basil leaves
- Extra virgin olive oil
- Balsamic glaze (optional)
- Salt and pepper to taste

Instructions:
1. Arrange the tomato slices and fresh mozzarella slices alternately on a serving platter.

2. Tuck fresh basil leaves in between the tomato and mozzarella slices.

3. Drizzle extra virgin olive oil over the salad.

4. Optionally, drizzle balsamic glaze over the salad for added sweetness and flavor.

5. Season with salt and pepper to taste.

6. Serve immediately and enjoy your delicious and vibrant Caprese salad!

This salad is best enjoyed fresh and at room temperature. It's a perfect appetizer or side dish, especially during the summer when tomatoes and basil are in season.

20. Mushroom risotto

Ingredients:
- 1 1/2 cups Arborio rice
- 4 cups vegetable broth, kept warm
- 2 tablespoons olive oil
- 1 onion, finely chopped
- 2 cloves garlic, minced
- 8 oz (225g) mushrooms (such as cremini or button), sliced
- 1/2 cup dry white wine (optional)
- 1/2 cup grated Parmesan cheese
- Salt and pepper to taste
- Fresh parsley, chopped, for garnish (optional)

Instructions:

1. In a large skillet or saucepan, heat the olive oil over medium heat. Add the chopped onion and cook until softened, about 5 minutes.

2. Add the minced garlic to the skillet and cook for another minute until fragrant.

3. Add the sliced mushrooms to the skillet and cook until they release their moisture and start to brown, about 5-7 minutes.

4. Stir in the Arborio rice and cook for 1-2 minutes, stirring constantly, until the rice is coated with the oil and slightly translucent.

5. If using, pour in the white wine and stir until it has evaporated.

6. Begin adding the warm vegetable broth to the skillet, one ladleful at a time, stirring frequently and allowing each addition to be absorbed before adding more. Continue this process until the rice is creamy and cooked to your desired consistency, about 20-25 minutes.

7. Stir in the grated Parmesan cheese until melted and well combined.

8. Season the risotto with salt and pepper to taste.

9. Remove the risotto from heat and let it sit for a minute or two to thicken.

10. Serve the mushroom risotto hot, garnished with chopped fresh parsley if desired.

11. Enjoy your creamy and flavorful mushroom risotto!

This dish is perfect as a comforting main course or as a side dish for a special meal. The creamy texture and earthy flavor of the mushrooms make it a true delight for the taste buds.

21. Spinach and cheese stuffed shells

Ingredients:
- 1 box jumbo pasta shells
- 2 tbsp olive oil
- 1 onion, chopped
- 3 cloves garlic, minced
- 10 oz fresh spinach, chopped
- 1 container ricotta cheese
- 1 cup shredded mozzarella cheese
- 1/2 cup grated Parmesan cheese
- 1 large egg
- 1 tsp dried Italian seasoning
- Salt and pepper to taste
- 2 cups marinara sauce

Instructions:
1. Cook pasta shells according to package instructions, then set aside.

2. Sauté onion and garlic in olive oil until softened.

3. Add spinach and cook until wilted.

4. In a bowl, mix ricotta, mozzarella, Parmesan, egg, Italian seasoning, salt, and pepper.

5. Combine spinach mixture with cheese mixture.

6. Stuff pasta shells with mixture and place in a baking dish.

7. Cover with marinara sauce and extra Parmesan.

8. Bake at 375°F (190°C) for 25-30 mins covered, then 5-10 mins uncovered.

9. Garnish with basil or parsley if desired.

10. Serve and enjoy your stuffed shells!

This version maintains all the essential steps and flavors while being more concise.

22. Tofu stir-fry with broccoli and carrots

Ingredients:
- 14 oz (400g) firm tofu, pressed and cubed
- 2 tablespoons soy sauce or tamari
- 1 tablespoon cornstarch
- 2 tablespoons vegetable oil
- 2 cups broccoli florets
- 1 cup sliced carrots
- 2 cloves garlic, minced
- 1 tablespoon grated ginger
- 1/4 cup vegetable broth or water
- Salt and pepper to taste
- Cooked rice for serving

Instructions:
1. In a bowl, toss the tofu cubes with soy sauce (or tamari) until evenly coated. Sprinkle cornstarch over the tofu and toss again until coated.

2. Heat 1 tablespoon of vegetable oil in a large skillet or wok over medium-high heat. Add the tofu cubes and cook until golden brown and crispy on all sides, about 5-7 minutes. Remove tofu from the skillet and set aside.

3. In the same skillet, add the remaining tablespoon of vegetable oil. Add minced garlic and grated ginger, and cook for about 1 minute until fragrant.

4. Add broccoli florets and sliced carrots to the skillet. Stir-fry for about 3-4 minutes until vegetables are crisp-tender.

5. Return the cooked tofu to the skillet. Pour vegetable broth (or water) over the tofu and vegetables. Stir to combine.

6. Cook for another 1-2 minutes until heated through and the sauce has thickened slightly.

7. Season with salt and pepper to taste.

8. Serve the tofu stir-fry with broccoli and carrots over cooked rice.

9. Enjoy your delicious and nutritious stir-fry!

This tofu stir-fry is a quick and healthy meal that's perfect for busy weeknights. It's packed with protein and veggies, and the savory sauce adds delicious flavor.

23. Quinoa stuffed peppers

Ingredients:
- 4 large bell peppers
- 1 cup quinoa
- 2 cups vegetable broth
- 1 tbsp olive oil
- 1 onion, diced
- 2 cloves garlic, minced
- 1 zucchini, diced
- 1 cup corn kernels
- 1 can (14 oz) black beans, drained
- 1 tsp ground cumin
- 1 tsp chili powder
- Salt and pepper to taste
- 1 cup shredded cheese
- Fresh cilantro or parsley for garnish
- Optional: avocado slices, sour cream or Greek yogurt for serving

Instructions:
1. Preheat oven to 375°F (190°C). Grease a baking dish.

2. Cut tops off peppers, remove seeds and membranes, and place in the baking dish.

3. Cook quinoa in vegetable broth, then set aside.

4. Sauté onion and garlic in olive oil. Add zucchini, corn, black beans, cumin, and chili powder. Cook until tender.

5. Stir in cooked quinoa. Season with salt and pepper.

6. Fill peppers with quinoa mixture, top with cheese.

7. Bake covered for 25-30 minutes, then uncovered for 5 minutes until cheese is melted.

8. Garnish with cilantro or parsley.

9. Serve with optional avocado slices and sour cream or Greek yogurt.

10. Enjoy your delicious quinoa stuffed peppers!

This version retains all the essential steps and flavors while being more concise.

24. Eggplant rollatini

Ingredients:
- 2 medium eggplants, thinly sliced lengthwise
- Salt
- Olive oil for brushing
- 2 cups marinara sauce
- 1 cup ricotta cheese
- 1 cup shredded mozzarella cheese
- 1/2 cup grated Parmesan cheese
- 1 large egg
- 1 teaspoon dried Italian seasoning
- Fresh basil leaves for garnish (optional)

Instructions:
1. Preheat your oven to 375°F (190°C). Line a baking sheet with parchment paper.

2. Lay the eggplant slices on the prepared baking sheet in a single layer. Sprinkle both sides with salt and let them sit for about 15 minutes to draw out excess moisture.

3. After 15 minutes, pat the eggplant slices dry with paper towels to remove the excess salt and moisture.

4. Brush both sides of the eggplant slices with olive oil. Place them back on the baking sheet.

5. Bake the eggplant slices in the preheated oven for about 10-12 minutes, or until they are soft and pliable. Remove from the oven and let them cool slightly.

6. In a mixing bowl, combine ricotta cheese, shredded mozzarella cheese, grated Parmesan cheese, egg, and dried Italian seasoning. Mix until well combined.

7. Spread a thin layer of marinara sauce in the bottom of a baking dish. Place a spoonful of the cheese mixture onto each eggplant slice and roll it up.

8. Place the rolled eggplant slices seam side down in the baking dish. Spoon the remaining marinara sauce over the top of the rolled eggplant slices.

9. Sprinkle additional shredded mozzarella cheese and grated Parmesan cheese over the top. Bake in the preheated oven for 20-25 minutes, or until the cheese is melted and bubbly.

10. Remove from the oven and let it cool for a few minutes before serving. Garnish with fresh basil leaves if desired. Serve your delicious eggplant rollatini hot and enjoy!

25. Roasted vegetable medley

Ingredients:
- 2 cups cherry tomatoes, halved
- 2 bell peppers, diced
- 1 red onion, sliced
- 2 zucchinis, sliced
- 1 eggplant, diced
- 3 tablespoons olive oil
- 2 cloves garlic, minced
- 1 teaspoon dried thyme
- 1 teaspoon dried rosemary
- Salt and pepper to taste
- Fresh parsley for garnish (optional)

Instructions:
1. Preheat your oven to 400°F (200°C). Line a baking sheet with parchment paper or aluminum foil.

2. In a large bowl, combine the cherry tomatoes, diced bell peppers, sliced red onion, sliced zucchinis, and diced eggplant.

3. Drizzle olive oil over the vegetables and toss to coat evenly.

4. Sprinkle minced garlic, dried thyme, dried rosemary, salt, and pepper over the vegetables. Toss again to distribute the seasonings.

5. Spread the seasoned vegetables out in an even layer on the prepared baking sheet.

6. Roast in the preheated oven for 25-30 minutes, stirring halfway through cooking, until the vegetables are tender and caramelized.

7. Once done, remove the roasted vegetable medley from the oven and transfer to a serving dish.

8. Garnish with fresh parsley if desired. Serve hot and enjoy your delicious and colorful roasted vegetable medley!

This roasted vegetable medley is versatile and can be customized with your favorite vegetables and seasonings. It's a simple and nutritious side dish that pairs well with any main course.

26. Baked tofu with herbs

Ingredients:
- 1 block (14 oz / 400g) firm tofu, drained and pressed
- 2 tablespoons olive oil
- 2 cloves garlic, minced
- 1 tablespoon chopped fresh herbs (such as rosemary, thyme, or parsley)
- 1 tablespoon soy sauce or tamari
- Salt and pepper to taste

Instructions:
1. Preheat your oven to 375°F (190°C). Line a baking sheet with parchment paper or aluminum foil.

2. Cut the pressed tofu into cubes or slices, depending on your preference.

3. In a small bowl, whisk together the olive oil, minced garlic, chopped fresh herbs, soy sauce (or tamari), salt, and pepper.

4. Place the tofu cubes or slices in a single layer on the prepared baking sheet.

5. Pour the herb and olive oil mixture over the tofu, making sure each piece is coated evenly.

6. Bake in the preheated oven for 25-30 minutes, flipping halfway through cooking, until the tofu is golden brown and crispy on the outside.

7. Once done, remove the baked tofu from the oven and let it cool for a few minutes before serving.

8. Serve hot as a main course or as a protein-rich addition to salads, bowls, or sandwiches.

9. Enjoy your delicious and flavorful baked tofu with herbs!

This baked tofu is simple to prepare and bursting with flavor from the fresh herbs and garlic. It's a versatile dish that can be enjoyed on its own or incorporated into a variety of dishes.

27. Vegetable fajitas with guacamole

Ingredients:
- 2 bell peppers, sliced
- 1 onion, sliced
- 1 zucchini, sliced
- 1 yellow squash, sliced
- 2 tbsp olive oil
- 1 tbsp chili powder
- 1 tsp ground cumin
- 1 tsp paprika
- Salt and pepper to taste
- 8 small flour tortillas
- Optional toppings: salsa, sour cream, shredded cheese, chopped cilantro

Instructions:
1. Toss sliced vegetables with olive oil, chili powder, cumin, paprika, salt, and pepper.

2. Roast at 400°F (200°C) for 20-25 minutes until tender.

3. Warm tortillas.

4. Serve vegetables with tortillas and optional toppings.

Guacamole:
Ingredients:
- 2 ripe avocados, peeled and pitted
- 1/4 cup diced onion
- 1/4 cup diced tomato
- 1 tbsp chopped cilantro
- 1 tbsp lime juice
- 1/2 tsp minced garlic
- Salt and pepper to taste

Instructions:
1. Mash avocados, then mix in onion, tomato, cilantro, lime juice, garlic, salt, and pepper.

2. Adjust seasoning if needed.

3. Serve immediately or refrigerate until ready to use.

28. Lentil salad with lemon vinaigrette

Ingredients:
- 1 cup dry green or brown lentils
- 2 cups water or vegetable broth
- 1/4 cup chopped red onion
- 1/4 cup chopped bell pepper (any color)
- 1/4 cup chopped cucumber
- 1/4 cup chopped cherry tomatoes
- 2 tablespoons chopped fresh parsley
- Salt and pepper to taste

Lemon Vinaigrette:
- 3 tablespoons extra virgin olive oil
- 2 tablespoons freshly squeezed lemon juice
- 1 teaspoon Dijon mustard
- 1 teaspoon honey or maple syrup (optional)
- Salt and pepper to taste

Instructions:
1. Rinse the lentils under cold water. In a medium saucepan, bring water or vegetable broth to a boil. Add the lentils, reduce heat to low, cover, and simmer for 15-20 minutes, or until the lentils are tender but still hold their shape. Drain any excess liquid and let the lentils cool slightly.

2. In a large bowl, combine the cooked lentils, chopped red onion, bell pepper, cucumber, cherry tomatoes, and fresh parsley. Season with salt and pepper to taste.

3. In a small bowl, whisk together the extra virgin olive oil, lemon juice, Dijon mustard, honey or maple syrup (if using), salt, and pepper until well combined.

4. Pour the lemon vinaigrette over the lentil salad and toss until everything is evenly coated.
5. Taste and adjust seasoning if necessary.

6. Serve the lentil salad immediately, or refrigerate for a few hours to allow the flavors to meld together before serving.

This lentil salad with lemon vinaigrette is refreshing, nutritious, and bursting with flavor. It's perfect as a side dish or a light meal on its own. Enjoy!

29. Roasted beet and goat cheese salad

Ingredients:
- 4 medium beets, peeled and sliced
- 2 tablespoons olive oil
- Salt and pepper to taste
- 4 cups mixed salad greens (such as arugula, spinach, or mixed greens)
- 1/4 cup crumbled goat cheese
- 1/4 cup chopped walnuts or pecans (optional)
- Balsamic glaze for drizzling (optional)

Instructions:
1. Preheat your oven to 400°F (200°C). Line a baking sheet with parchment paper.

2. Place the peeled and sliced beets on the prepared baking sheet. Drizzle with olive oil and season with salt and pepper to taste. Toss to coat evenly.

3. Roast the beets in the preheated oven for 25-30 minutes, or until tender and caramelized, flipping halfway through cooking.

4. While the beets are roasting, prepare the salad greens in a large bowl.

5. Once the beets are done, let them cool slightly before adding them to the salad greens.

6. Sprinkle crumbled goat cheese and chopped walnuts or pecans (if using) over the salad.

7. Drizzle with balsamic glaze for extra flavor (if desired).

8. Toss the salad gently to combine all the ingredients.

9. Serve immediately and enjoy your delicious roasted beet and goat cheese salad!

This salad is perfect as a side dish or a light meal. The combination of sweet roasted beets, creamy goat cheese, and crunchy nuts creates a wonderful flavor and texture contrast.

30. Broccoli and cheese stuffed potatoes

Ingredients:
- 4 large russet potatoes
- 2 cups broccoli florets, chopped
- 1 cup shredded cheddar cheese
- 1/2 cup sour cream
- 2 tablespoons butter
- Salt and pepper to taste
- Chopped chives or green onions for garnish (optional)

Instructions:
1. Preheat your oven to 400°F (200°C). Scrub the potatoes clean and pierce them several times with a fork.

2. Place the potatoes directly on the oven rack and bake for 45-60 minutes, or until tender when pierced with a fork.

3. While the potatoes are baking, steam or boil the broccoli florets until tender, about 5 minutes. Drain well and set aside.

4. Once the potatoes are done, remove them from the oven and let them cool slightly.

5. Cut a slit lengthwise across the top of each potato, then gently squeeze the ends to open them up.

6. Scoop out the flesh from the potatoes into a large bowl, leaving a thin layer of potato inside the skins.

7. Mash the potato flesh with butter until smooth. Stir in the shredded cheddar cheese, sour cream, and steamed broccoli. Season with salt and pepper to taste.

8. Spoon the broccoli and cheese mixture back into the potato skins.

9. Place the stuffed potatoes on a baking sheet and return them to the oven. Bake for an additional 10-15 minutes, or until the cheese is melted and bubbly.

10. Remove from the oven and garnish with chopped chives or green onions if desired. Serve hot and enjoy your delicious broccoli and cheese stuffed potatoes!

These stuffed potatoes make for a satisfying and comforting meal. They're perfect for lunch or dinner, and you can customize them with your favorite toppings or add-ins.

31. Vegetarian chili

Ingredients:
- 2 tablespoons olive oil
- 1 onion, chopped
- 3 cloves garlic, minced
- 1 bell pepper, diced
- 1 zucchini, diced
- 1 carrot, diced
- 1 cup corn kernels
 (fresh, frozen, or canned)
- 2 cans (14 oz / 400g each)
diced tomatoes
- 1 can (14 oz / 400g) kidney
beans, drained and rinsed
- 1 can (14 oz / 400g) black
beans, drained and rinsed
- 2 tablespoons tomato paste
- 2 teaspoons chili powder
- 1 teaspoon ground cumin
- 1 teaspoon smoked paprika
- Salt and pepper to taste
- Optional toppings: shredded
cheese, sour cream, chopped
cilantro, sliced green onions,
avocado

Instructions:
1. Heat olive oil in a large pot over medium heat. Add chopped onion and cook until softened, about 5 minutes.

2. Add minced garlic and diced bell pepper to the pot. Cook for another 2-3 minutes until fragrant.

3. Stir in diced zucchini, diced carrot, and corn kernels. Cook for 5 minutes until vegetables start to soften.

4. Add diced tomatoes, drained and rinsed kidney beans, drained and rinsed black beans, tomato paste, chili powder, ground cumin, smoked paprika, salt, and pepper to the pot. Stir to combine.

5. Bring the chili to a simmer, then reduce heat to low. Cover and let it simmer for 20-30 minutes, stirring occasionally, until the vegetables are tender and the flavors are well combined.

6. Taste and adjust seasoning if necessary.

7. Serve the vegetarian chili hot, garnished with your favorite toppings. Enjoy your hearty and flavorful vegetarian chili!

This vegetarian chili is packed with protein and fiber from the beans and vegetables, making it a nutritious and satisfying meal. It's perfect for a cozy dinner or for meal prep to enjoy throughout the week.

32. Spinach and mushroom lasagna

Ingredients:
- 9 lasagna noodles
- 2 tbsp olive oil
- 1 onion, diced
- 3 cloves garlic, minced
- 8 oz mushrooms, sliced
- 6 cups fresh spinach leaves
- 2 cups ricotta cheese
- 1 cup shredded mozzarella cheese
- 1/2 cup grated Parmesan cheese
- 1 egg
- 1 tsp dried oregano
- 1 tsp dried basil
- Salt and pepper to taste
- 3 cups marinara sauce

Instructions:
1. Cook lasagna noodles according to package instructions.

2. Sauté onion and garlic, then add mushrooms and spinach until wilted.

3. Mix ricotta, mozzarella, Parmesan, egg, oregano, basil, salt, and pepper.

4. Layer marinara, noodles, ricotta mixture, mushroom-spinach mix, repeat.

5. Top with remaining sauce and cheeses.

6. Bake covered at 375°F (190°C) for 30 minutes, then uncovered for 10-15 minutes.

7. Let cool slightly before serving.

Enjoy your tasty spinach and mushroom lasagna!

33. Cauliflower fried rice

Ingredients:
- 1 head cauliflower, grated or finely chopped
- 2 tablespoons sesame oil or vegetable oil
- 2 cloves garlic, minced
- 1 onion, diced
- 1 carrot, diced
- 1/2 cup frozen peas
- 2 eggs, lightly beaten
- 3 tablespoons soy sauce or tamari
- 2 green onions, chopped
- Salt and pepper to taste
- Optional: cooked chicken, shrimp, or tofu for protein

Instructions:
1. In a large skillet or wok, heat sesame oil over medium heat.

2. Add minced garlic and diced onion to the skillet. Sauté until fragrant and onions are translucent, about 2-3 minutes.

3. Add diced carrot and frozen peas to the skillet. Cook until vegetables are tender, about 3-4 minutes.

4. Push the vegetables to one side of the skillet and pour the beaten eggs into the empty side. Let them cook for a minute until they start to set, then scramble them with a spatula until cooked through.

5. Add grated or finely chopped cauliflower to the skillet. Stir to combine with the cooked vegetables and eggs.

6. Pour soy sauce or tamari over the cauliflower mixture. Stir well to evenly distribute the sauce.

7. Cook for another 5-7 minutes, stirring occasionally, until the cauliflower is cooked through and slightly crispy.

8. Season with salt and pepper to taste. If using, add cooked chicken, shrimp, or tofu to the skillet and toss to combine.

9. Remove from heat and garnish with chopped green onions before serving. Enjoy your delicious and healthy cauliflower fried rice!

34. Tofu scramble with vegetables

Ingredients:
- 1 block (14 oz / 400g) firm tofu, drained and crumbled
- 2 tablespoons olive oil
- 1 onion, diced
- 2 cloves garlic, minced
- 1 bell pepper, diced
- 1 cup diced mushrooms
- 1 cup baby spinach leaves
- 1 teaspoon ground turmeric
- 1/2 teaspoon ground cumin
- 1/2 teaspoon paprika
- Salt and pepper to taste
- Optional toppings: chopped fresh herbs (such as parsley or cilantro), sliced avocado, salsa

Instructions:
1. Heat olive oil in a large skillet over medium heat.

2. Add diced onion and minced garlic to the skillet. Sauté until softened and fragrant, about 3-4 minutes.

3. Add diced bell pepper and mushrooms to the skillet. Cook until vegetables are tender, about 5-7 minutes.

4. Add crumbled tofu to the skillet, along with ground turmeric, ground cumin, paprika, salt, and pepper. Stir well to combine.

5. Cook tofu mixture for another 5-7 minutes, stirring occasionally, until heated through and slightly golden.

6. Add baby spinach leaves to the skillet and cook until wilted, about 2 minutes.

7. Taste and adjust seasoning if necessary.

8. Remove from heat and serve the tofu scramble hot. Garnish with chopped fresh herbs, sliced avocado, and salsa if desired. Enjoy your flavorful and nutritious tofu scramble with vegetables!

This tofu scramble is a delicious and satisfying breakfast or brunch option that's packed with protein and veggies. It's also versatile, so feel free to customize it with your favorite vegetables and seasonings.

35. Butternut squash soup

Ingredients:
- 1 medium butternut squash, peeled, seeded, and diced (about 4 cups)
- 1 tablespoon olive oil
- 1 onion, diced
- 2 cloves garlic, minced
- 4 cups vegetable broth
- 1 teaspoon ground cumin
- 1/2 teaspoon ground cinnamon
- Salt and pepper to taste
- Optional garnish: fresh parsley, cream, toasted pumpkin seeds

Instructions:
1. Heat olive oil in a large pot over medium heat.

2. Add diced onion and minced garlic to the pot. Sauté until softened and fragrant, about 3-4 minutes.

3. Add diced butternut squash to the pot. Cook for another 5-7 minutes, stirring occasionally, until slightly caramelized.

4. Pour vegetable broth into the pot, making sure the squash is mostly covered. Bring to a boil, then reduce heat to low and simmer for about 20-25 minutes, or until the squash is tender.

5. Using an immersion blender or a regular blender, puree the soup until smooth and creamy. Be careful when blending hot liquids.

6. Stir in ground cumin and ground cinnamon. Season with salt and pepper to taste.

7. If the soup is too thick, you can add more vegetable broth or water to reach your desired consistency.

8. Taste and adjust seasoning if necessary.

9. Ladle the butternut squash soup into bowls and garnish with fresh parsley, a drizzle of cream, and toasted pumpkin seeds if desired. Serve hot and enjoy your comforting and flavorful butternut squash soup!

This soup is perfect for chilly days and makes for a cozy and nutritious meal. Plus, it's easy to make and can be customized with your favorite herbs and spices.

36. Stuffed cabbage rolls with rice and lentils

Ingredients:
- 1 large head cabbage
- 1 cup cooked rice
- 1 cup cooked lentils
- 1 onion, finely chopped
- 2 cloves garlic, minced
- 1 carrot, grated
- 1 celery stalk, finely chopped
- 1 tbsp olive oil
- 1 tsp dried thyme
- 1 tsp dried oregano
- Salt and pepper to taste
- 2 cups marinara sauce
- Optional: shredded cheese for topping

Instructions:

1. Precook cabbage in boiling water, remove leaves, and let cool.

2. Sauté onion, garlic, carrot, and celery in olive oil until softened.

3. Mix cooked rice, lentils, sautéed vegetables, thyme, oregano, salt, and pepper.

4. Fill cabbage leaves with rice-lentil mixture, roll tightly.

5. Place cabbage rolls in a greased baking dish.

6. Cover with marinara sauce, bake at 375°F (190°C) for 45-50 minutes.

7. Optionally, add shredded cheese during the last 10 minutes of baking.

8. Serve hot.

Enjoy your tasty stuffed cabbage rolls with rice and lentils!

37. Greek stuffed tomatoes with rice and herbs

Ingredients:
- 6 large tomatoes
- 1 cup uncooked long-grain white rice
- 1/2 cup chopped fresh parsley
- 1/4 cup chopped fresh dill
- 2 tablespoons chopped fresh mint
- 1 onion, finely chopped
- 2 cloves garlic, minced
- 1/4 cup olive oil
- Juice of 1 lemon
- Salt and pepper to taste
- Crumbled feta cheese for topping (optional)

Instructions:

1. Cut the tops off the tomatoes and scoop out the insides, reserving the pulp. Chop the pulp.

2. In a bowl, combine the chopped tomato pulp, rice, parsley, dill, mint, onion, garlic, olive oil, lemon juice, salt, and pepper. Mix well.

3. Stuff the tomato shells with the rice mixture, packing it in tightly.

4. Place the stuffed tomatoes in a baking dish. If desired, top with crumbled feta cheese.

5. Bake at 375°F for 45-60 minutes, until the rice is tender and the tomatoes are softened.

6. Serve warm or at room temperature. Enjoy!

38. Vegetable paella

Ingredients:
- 3 tablespoons olive oil
- 1 onion, diced
- 3 cloves garlic, minced
- 1 red bell pepper, diced
- 2 cups short grain Spanish rice
- 1 teaspoon smoked paprika
- 1/2 teaspoon saffron threads (or 1/4 tsp ground turmeric)
- 4 cups vegetable or faux chicken broth
- 1 cup frozen peas
- 1 cup diced tomatoes
- 1 cup artichoke hearts, quartered
- Salt and pepper to taste
- Chopped parsley for garnish

Instructions:

1. Heat the olive oil in a large skillet or paella pan over medium-high heat. Add the onions and sauté for 2-3 minutes until translucent.

2. Add the garlic and bell pepper and cook for 1 minute until fragrant.

3. Stir in the rice and smoked paprika to coat the rice with oil. Cook for 2-3 minutes, stirring frequently.

4. Add the saffron threads and vegetable broth. Bring to a simmer.

5. Reduce heat to medium-low, cover and cook for 15 minutes.

6. Remove lid and arrange peas, tomatoes, and artichokes on top of the rice.

7. Cover and cook for 5-10 more minutes until rice is tender and liquid is absorbed.

8. Remove from heat and let stand covered for 5 minutes.

9. Season with salt and pepper to taste. Garnish with chopped parsley.

39. Spinach and artichoke dip with whole grain crackers

Ingredients:
- 1 (10 oz) package frozen chopped spinach, thawed and drained
- 1 (14 oz) can artichoke hearts, drained and chopped
- 1 cup shredded mozzarella cheese
- 1/2 cup grated parmesan cheese
- 1/2 cup mayonnaise
- 1/2 cup sour cream
- 3 cloves garlic, minced
- 1 tsp lemon juice
- 1/4 tsp red pepper flakes (optional)
- Salt and pepper to taste
- Whole grain crackers, for serving

Instructions:
1. Preheat oven to 350°F (175°C). Grease a baking dish.

2. In a large bowl, mix together the spinach, artichoke hearts, mozzarella, parmesan, mayonnaise, sour cream, garlic, lemon juice, red pepper flakes if using, and salt and pepper until well combined.

3. Transfer the dip mixture to the prepared baking dish and spread it out evenly.

4. Bake for 20-25 minutes, until heated through and cheese is melted and lightly browned on top.

5. Remove from oven and let cool for 5 minutes before serving.

6. Serve hot with whole grain crackers for dipping. You can also serve with bread, tortilla chips, or fresh veggies.

Some tips:
- Squeeze excess moisture out of thawed spinach before adding to prevent a watery dip.
- Use marinated artichoke hearts for extra flavor.
- Add some shredded cheddar in addition to the mozzarella for a cheese blend.
- For a lighter dip, use low-fat mayo, sour cream and cheese.

40. Baked falafel with tzatziki sauce

Ingredients:
- 1 cup dried chickpeas,
  soaked overnight and drained
- 1 onion, roughly chopped
- 4 cloves garlic, minced
- 1 cup fresh parsley, chopped
- 1 cup fresh cilantro, chopped
- 1 tsp ground cumin
- 1 tsp ground coriander
- 1 tsp baking soda
- 1/2 tsp salt
- 1/4 tsp black pepper
- 2 tbsp all-purpose flour
- Olive oil cooking spray

Tzatziki Sauce:
- 1 cup Greek yogurt
- 1/2 cucumber, grated and
drained of excess moisture
- 2 cloves garlic, minced
- 2 tbsp fresh dill, chopped
- 1 tbsp lemon juice
- 1/2 tsp salt

Instructions:

1. In a food processor, pulse the chickpeas until broken down but still slightly chunky. Transfer to a bowl.

2. Add the onion, garlic, parsley, cilantro, spices, baking soda, salt, pepper and flour to the chickpeas and mix well until fully combined.

3. Form the mixture into ping pong sized balls and place on a baking sheet lined with parchment paper. Spray the tops with olive oil cooking spray.

4. Bake at 400°F for 20-25 minutes, flipping halfway, until golden brown and crispy on the outside.

5. While the falafel bakes, make the tzatziki sauce by mixing together the yogurt, grated cucumber, garlic, dill, lemon juice and salt. Refrigerate until ready to serve.

6. Serve the warm baked falafel balls with the cool tzatziki sauce on the side for dipping. You can stuff them into pita breads with toppings like tomato, lettuce and red onion for a portable meal.

The baking method keeps the falafel crispy on the outside while keeping the interior moist. The bright, herby tzatziki sauce makes the perfect cooling accompaniment. Enjoy!

41. Lentil burgers with whole grain buns

Ingredients:
- 1 cup dried green or brown lentils, rinsed
- 3 cups vegetable broth or water
- 1 tablespoon olive oil
- 1 onion, finely chopped
- 2 garlic cloves, minced
- 1 carrot, grated
- 1 cup breadcrumbs (preferably whole wheat)
- 1/4 cup fresh parsley, chopped
- 1 teaspoon cumin
- 1 teaspoon smoked paprika
- Salt and pepper to taste
- Whole grain burger buns
- Desired toppings like lettuce, tomato, avocado, etc.

Instructions:

1. In a saucepan, combine the lentils and vegetable broth/water. Bring to a boil, then reduce heat and simmer for 20-25 minutes until lentils are tender but still hold their shape. Drain any excess liquid.

2. In a skillet, heat the olive oil over medium heat. Sauté the onion and garlic until translucent, about 3-4 minutes.

3. In a large bowl, mash about 3/4 of the cooked lentils with a potato masher or fork, leaving some lentils whole for texture.

4. Add the sautéed onion/garlic, grated carrot, breadcrumbs, parsley, cumin, smoked paprika, and salt and pepper. Mix until well combined.

5. Form the lentil mixture into patties, about 1/2 cup of mixture per patty.

6. Heat a skillet over medium heat and cook the patties for 3-4 minutes per side until browned and heated through.

7. Serve the warm lentil patties on whole grain buns topped with desired toppings like lettuce, tomato, avocado, etc.

The lentils pack these veggie burgers with protein, fiber and nutrients. The whole grain buns add heartiness. You can make the patties ahead of time and refrigerate or freeze for easy meals. Serve with a salad or baked fries for a satisfying meatless meal!

42. Ratatouille tart

Ingredients:
- 1 sheet frozen puff pastry, thawed
- 1 eggplant, sliced into 1/4 inch rounds
- 1 zucchini, sliced into 1/4 inch rounds
- 1 yellow squash, sliced into 1/4 inch rounds
- 1 red bell pepper, sliced
- 1 yellow onion, thinly sliced
- 4 cloves garlic, minced
- 2 tablespoons olive oil
- 1 teaspoon dried thyme
- Salt and pepper to taste
- 1 egg, beaten with 1 tbsp water (for egg wash)
- 1/2 cup shredded cheese (gruyere, mozzarella or provolone)

Instructions:

1. Preheat oven to 400°F (200°C). Roll out the puff pastry into a 10-inch square on a parchment lined baking sheet. Score a 1-inch border around the edges with a knife (without cutting all the way through). Prick the center area with a fork. Bake for 15 minutes until lightly golden. Allow to cool slightly.

2. In a bowl, toss the sliced eggplant, zucchini, squash, pepper and onion with olive oil, garlic, thyme, salt and pepper.

3. Arrange the vegetable slices in an alternating pattern on the baked puff pastry, staying within the scored border.

4. Brush the borders of the pastry with the egg wash. Sprinkle the shredded cheese over the arranged vegetables.

5. Bake for 20-25 minutes until the vegetables are tender and the pastry is golden brown.

6. Allow to cool slightly before slicing and serving. Can be served warm or at room temperature.

This colorful ratatouille tart makes a stunning vegetarian main or appetizer. The flaky puff pastry base holds the layered roasted veggies perfectly. You can also add marinara sauce or pesto dolloped over the top. Enjoy!

43. Vegetable curry with coconut milk

Ingredients:
- 2 tablespoons olive oil or coconut oil
- 1 onion, diced
- 3 cloves garlic, minced
- 1 tablespoon grated fresh ginger
- 2 tablespoons curry powder
- 1 teaspoon ground cumin
- 1/2 teaspoon ground coriander
- 1/4 teaspoon cayenne pepper
(or more to taste)
- 1 (14 oz) can diced tomatoes
- 1 (14 oz) can coconut milk
- 1 cup vegetable or chicken broth
- 1 potato, peeled and cubed
- 2 carrots, peeled and sliced
- 1 bell pepper, diced
- 1 cup cauliflower florets
- 1 cup green beans, trimmed and
cut into 1-inch pieces
- Salt and pepper to taste
- Fresh cilantro for garnish

Instructions:
1. In a large pot, heat the oil over medium heat. Add the onions and sauté for 2-3 minutes until translucent.

2. Add the garlic and ginger, cook for 1 minute until fragrant.

3. Stir in the curry powder, cumin, coriander and cayenne. Toast the spices for 30 seconds.

4. Pour in the diced tomatoes, coconut milk and broth. Add the potato, carrots, bell pepper, cauliflower and green beans.

5. Season with salt and pepper to taste.

6. Bring to a boil, then reduce heat and let simmer for 20-25 minutes, until vegetables are fork-tender.

7. Adjust seasoning if needed, adding more salt, pepper or cayenne for heat.

8. Garnish with fresh cilantro. Serve over basmati rice or with naan bread.

This fragrant coconut vegetable curry is hearty, nutritious and full of flavor from the spice blend and creamy coconut milk. You can mix and match whatever veggies you have on hand like chickpeas, spinach or zucchini. For a protein boost, add some cooked chicken or tofu. Enjoy!

44. Stuffed mushrooms with spinach and cheese

Ingredients:
- 24 large mushroom caps (stems removed and chopped)
- 2 tablespoons olive oil, plus more for brushing
- 1 shallot, finely chopped
- 3 garlic cloves, minced
- 10 oz frozen chopped spinach, thawed and drained of excess moisture
- 1/2 cup ricotta cheese
- 1/2 cup shredded mozzarella cheese
- 1/3 cup grated parmesan cheese
- 1 egg, lightly beaten
- 1/4 teaspoon red pepper flakes (optional)
- Salt and pepper to taste

Instructions:

1. Preheat oven to 400°F (200°C). Brush the mushroom caps lightly with olive oil on both sides and place cap-side up on a baking sheet.

2. In a skillet, heat 2 tbsp olive oil over medium heat. Sauté the chopped mushroom stems and shallot for 3-4 minutes until softened.

3. Add the minced garlic and sauté for 1 minute until fragrant.

4. Add in the drained spinach and season with salt, pepper and red pepper flakes, if using. Cook for 2 minutes until heated through.

5. Remove spinach mixture from heat and let cool slightly. In a bowl, mix together the spinach, ricotta, mozzarella, parmesan and beaten egg until well combined.

6. Using a spoon or piping bag, generously stuff the mushroom caps with the spinach and cheese filling.

7. Bake for 15-18 minutes until the filling is hot and the cheese is melted and lightly browned on top.

8. Serve the stuffed mushrooms warm as an appetizer or vegetarian main course.

The savory filling with three cheeses, garlic and spinach is the perfect stuffing for tender mushroom caps. You can prep these ahead and bake just before serving. For extra presentation, you can remove the stems completely before stuffing. Enjoy!

45. Veggie sushi rolls with avocado and cucumber

Ingredients:
- 4 sheets sushi nori (seaweed wraps)
- 1 cup sushi rice, cooked per package instructions
- 1 avocado, sliced
- 1/2 English cucumber, sliced into strips
- 2 carrots, peeled into strips
- 1/2 red bell pepper, sliced into strips
- 2 tablespoons sesame seeds
- Soy sauce, pickled ginger and wasabi for serving

For the Rice:
- 1 cup sushi rice
- 1 cup water
- 2 tablespoons rice vinegar
- 1 tablespoon sugar
- 1/2 teaspoon salt

Instructions:

1. Cook the sushi rice according to package directions, then transfer to a bowl. Season with rice vinegar, sugar and salt. Allow to cool slightly.

2. Place a sushi mat or thin towel on a flat surface. Place one nori sheet shiny-side down on the mat.

3. With wet fingers or a rice paddle, spread 1/4 of the rice evenly over the nori sheet in a thin layer leaving a 1-inch border on the far side.

4. In the center of the rice, lay a few slices of avocado, cucumber strips, carrot strips and bell pepper strips horizontally.

5. Using the mat, carefully roll up the nori and rice tightly from the side closest to you, enclosing the filling. Roll all the way and seal the end with a little water.

6. Sprinkle the roll with sesame seeds and press gently to adhere.

7. With a very sharp knife, slice the roll into 6-8 pieces. Repeat with remaining ingredients to make 3 more rolls. Serve immediately with soy sauce, pickled ginger and wasabi for dipping.

For make-ahead, cover the rolls tightly with plastic wrap and refrigerate for up to 8 hours before slicing. These fresh veggie rolls are so flavorful and make a healthy vegetarian meal or appetizer. You can get creative with different veggie fillings you enjoy.

46. Quinoa tabbouleh

Ingredients:
- 1 cup quinoa, rinsed
- 1 3/4 cups water or vegetable broth
- 1 cup finely chopped parsley
- 1/2 cup finely chopped mint
- 1 cucumber, diced
- 2 tomatoes, diced
- 1/4 cup finely chopped red onion
- 3 tablespoons lemon juice
- 2 tablespoons olive oil
- 1 clove garlic, minced
- 1 teaspoon ground cumin
- Salt and pepper to taste

Instructions:

1. In a saucepan, combine the quinoa and water/broth. Bring to a boil, then reduce heat to low, cover and simmer for 15 minutes until liquid is absorbed.

2. Remove quinoa from heat and fluff with a fork. Allow to cool completely.

3. In a large bowl, mix together the cooled quinoa, chopped parsley, mint, cucumber, tomatoes and red onion.

4. In a small bowl, whisk together the lemon juice, olive oil, garlic, cumin and a pinch each of salt and pepper.

5. Pour the dressing over the quinoa salad and toss gently to combine all the ingredients.

6. Allow to sit for 30 minutes for the flavors to meld together before serving. Can be refrigerated for up to 3 days.

7. Garnish with extra chopped parsley and mint before serving, if desired.

The quinoa gives this classic Middle Eastern tabbouleh salad a protein boost, while maintaining the fresh herby flavor. It makes a light, flavorful vegetarian meal or side salad. You can also add crumbled feta or chickpeas for extra protein. Adjust lemon and seasonings to your taste preference. Enjoy!

47. Roasted Brussels sprouts with balsamic glaze

Ingredients:
- 1 cup quinoa, rinsed
- 1 3/4 cups water or vegetable broth
- 1 cup finely chopped parsley
- 1/2 cup finely chopped mint
- 1 cucumber, diced
- 2 tomatoes, diced
- 1/4 cup finely chopped red onion
- 3 tablespoons lemon juice
- 2 tablespoons olive oil
- 1 clove garlic, minced
- 1 teaspoon ground cumin
- Salt and pepper to taste

Instructions:

1. In a saucepan, combine the quinoa and water/broth. Bring to a boil, then reduce heat to low, cover and simmer for 15 minutes until liquid is absorbed.

2. Remove quinoa from heat and fluff with a fork. Allow to cool completely.

3. In a large bowl, mix together the cooled quinoa, chopped parsley, mint, cucumber, tomatoes and red onion.

4. In a small bowl, whisk together the lemon juice, olive oil, garlic, cumin and a pinch each of salt and pepper.

5. Pour the dressing over the quinoa salad and toss gently to combine all the ingredients.

6. Allow to sit for 30 minutes for the flavors to meld together before serving. Can be refrigerated for up to 3 days.

7. Garnish with extra chopped parsley and mint before serving, if desired.

The quinoa gives this classic Middle Eastern tabbouleh salad a protein boost, while maintaining the fresh herby flavor. It makes a light, flavorful vegetarian meal or side salad. You can also add crumbled feta or chickpeas for extra protein. Adjust lemon and seasonings to your taste preference. Enjoy!

48. Spinach and cheese stuffed mushrooms

Ingredients:
- 24 large mushroom caps, stems removed and chopped
- 2 tablespoons olive oil, divided
- 1 shallot, finely chopped
- 2 garlic cloves, minced
- 10 oz frozen chopped spinach, thawed and drained of excess moisture
- 1/2 cup ricotta cheese
- 1/2 cup shredded mozzarella cheese
- 1/4 cup grated parmesan cheese
- 1 egg, lightly beaten
- 1/4 teaspoon red pepper flakes (optional)
- Salt and pepper to taste

Instructions:

1. Preheat oven to 400°F (200°C). Brush the mushroom caps lightly with 1 tablespoon olive oil on both sides and place cap-side up on a baking sheet.

2. In a skillet, heat the remaining 1 tablespoon olive oil over medium heat. Sauté the chopped mushroom stems and shallot for 2-3 minutes until soft.

3. Add the garlic and sauté for 1 minute until fragrant.

4. Add the drained, thawed spinach and season with salt, pepper and red pepper flakes if using. Cook for 2 minutes.

5. Remove from heat and let cool slightly. In a bowl, mix the spinach mixture with the ricotta, mozzarella, parmesan and beaten egg until well combined.

6. Using a spoon or piping bag, generously stuff the mushroom caps with the spinach and cheese filling.

7. Bake for 15-18 minutes until the mushrooms are tender and the filling is hot and melted.

8. Serve the stuffed mushrooms warm as an appetizer or side dish.

These spinach and cheese stuffed mushrooms make such a flavorful vegetarian bite! The filling of creamy cheeses, garlic and spinach is the perfect savory stuffing for tender mushroom caps. You can prepare the filling ahead of time for easy assembly before baking. Enjoy!

49. Tofu and vegetable kebabs

Ingredients:
- 14 oz extra-firm tofu, drained and cubed
- 2 bell peppers (different colors), cut into 1-inch pieces
- 1 red onion, cut into 1-inch pieces
- 1 zucchini, sliced into rounds
- 8 oz mushrooms, left whole if small or halved
- 1 cup cherry tomatoes
- 1/4 cup olive oil
- 2 tablespoons soy sauce
- 1 tablespoon rice vinegar
- 2 cloves garlic, minced
- 1 teaspoon dried basil
- Salt and pepper to taste
- Metal or wooden skewers (if using wooden, soak in water for 30 mins)

Instructions:
1. In a shallow baking dish, whisk together the olive oil, soy sauce, rice vinegar, garlic, dried basil and a pinch each of salt and pepper.

2. Add the cubed tofu and toss gently to coat in the marinade. Let marinate for 30 minutes, tossing halfway.

3. Carefully thread the marinated tofu, bell peppers, red onion, zucchini, mushrooms and cherry tomatoes onto the skewers in an alternating pattern.

4. Preheat grill or grill pan to medium-high heat. Brush grates with oil.

5. Grill the skewers for 12-15 minutes, turning occasionally, until the vegetables are tender and the tofu is lightly charred.

6. Brush any remaining marinade over the skewers while grilling for extra flavor. Remove skewers from grill and let cool slightly before serving.

7. Serve the tofu and veggie skewers over rice or with a salad or pita bread. You can also serve with desired dipping sauces like teriyaki, peanut or tzatziki sauce.

These grilled tofu kebabs packed with colorful veggies make for a delicious and satisfying vegetarian meal. The tofu gets nicely charred on the outside while staying tender on the inside from the marinade. Feel free to mix up the vegetable varieties based on your preference. Enjoy!

50. Black bean and corn salad

Ingredients:
- 1 (15 oz) can black beans, rinsed and drained
- 1 (15 oz) can corn kernels, drained
- 1 red bell pepper, diced
- 1/2 red onion, diced
- 1 jalapeno, seeds removed and minced (optional for heat)
- 1/4 cup chopped fresh cilantro
- 2 tablespoons lime juice
- 2 tablespoons olive oil
- 1 teaspoon ground cumin
- 1 teaspoon chili powder
- Salt and pepper to taste

Instructions:

1. In a large bowl, combine the rinsed black beans, corn kernels, diced bell pepper, red onion, jalapeno (if using), and chopped cilantro.

2. In a small bowl, whisk together the lime juice, olive oil, cumin, chili powder, and a pinch each of salt and pepper.

3. Pour the dressing over the bean and corn mixture and toss gently to coat everything evenly.

4. Taste and adjust seasoning as needed, adding more lime juice for tang, salt and pepper for flavor, or jalapeno for heat.

5. Refrigerate for 30 minutes to allow flavors to meld before serving. Can be made a day ahead.

6. Serve chilled or at room temperature as a salad, dip or topping for tacos, burritos or salads.

This colorful black bean and corn salad is full of southwestern flavors from the lime, cumin, chili powder and fresh cilantro. It's a tasty protein-packed vegetarian dish that goes well as a salad, side or dip with some tortilla chips. You can also toss in some diced avocado right before serving for extra creaminess. Enjoy!

51. Lentil shepherd's pie

Ingredients:
- 1 cup dried green or brown lentils, rinsed
- 4 cups vegetable broth or water
- 2 tablespoons olive oil
- 1 onion, diced
- 2 carrots, peeled and diced
- 2 celery stalks, diced
- 3 cloves garlic, minced
- 1 tablespoon tomato paste
- 1 teaspoon dried thyme
- 1 teaspoon paprika
- Salt and pepper to taste
- 2 tablespoons all-purpose flour
- 1/2 cup frozen peas
- 4 cups mashed potatoes

Instructions:
1. In a saucepan, combine the lentils and broth/water. Bring to a boil, then reduce heat and simmer for 20-25 minutes until lentils are tender but still hold their shape. Drain any excess liquid.

2. In a skillet, heat the olive oil over medium heat. Sauté the onion, carrots and celery for 5-7 minutes until softened.

3. Add the garlic and cook for 1 minute until fragrant. Stir in the tomato paste, thyme, paprika and lentils. Season with salt and pepper.

4. Sprinkle in the flour and stir to coat vegetables. Cook for 2 minutes.

5. Stir in 1 cup of the cooked lentil cooking liquid to form a thick gravy. Add the peas.

6. Transfer the lentil mixture to a 9-inch pie plate or baking dish. Spread the mashed potatoes evenly over the top.

7. Use a fork to make decorative peaks on the mashed potato topping.

8. Bake at 400°F for 20-25 minutes until hot and the potatoes start to brown on the peaks. Allow to cool for 5 minutes before serving.

The hearty lentils simmered with savory vegetables make a perfect meat-free filling for this comfort food classic. You can use store-bought or homemade mashed potatoes on top. For extra richness, mix some cheese or cream into the potatoes before topping. Enjoy this nutritious and satisfying lentil shepherd's pie!

52. Stuffed artichokes with breadcrumbs and Parmesan

Ingredients:
- 4 large globe artichokes
- 1 lemon, halved
- 1 cup plain breadcrumbs
- 1/2 cup grated Parmesan cheese
- 1/4 cup chopped fresh parsley
- 2 garlic cloves, minced
- 1/2 tsp dried oregano
- 1/4 tsp salt
- 1/4 tsp black pepper
- 1/3 cup olive oil

Instructions:

1. Prepare the artichokes by cutting off the stem and top 1 inch of leaves. Use kitchen shears to trim off the sharp tips of the remaining leaves.

2. Rub all over with a lemon half to prevent browning.

3. In a pot of salted boiling water, parboil the artichokes for 15-20 minutes until the outer leaves can be easily pulled off. Drain upside down on a paper towel-lined plate.

4. In a bowl, mix together the breadcrumbs, Parmesan, parsley, garlic, oregano, salt, pepper and olive oil until well combined.

5. Gently spread apart the artichoke leaves and stuff the breadcrumb mixture into the center and between the leaves, pushing it in as you fan the leaves out.

6. Place the stuffed artichokes in a baking dish. Add 1/4 inch of water to the bottom of the dish.

7. Bake at 400°F for 20-25 minutes until the filling is golden brown and crispy on top. Serve the stuffed artichokes immediately while hot, squeezing fresh lemon juice over the top.

The tender artichoke leaves provide a perfect vessel for holding the savory, herbed breadcrumb and Parmesan stuffing. You can adjust ingredients like adding anchovies, sundried tomatoes or different herbs to the stuffing.

Let guests pull off the leaves and dip the bottoms into melted butter or marinara sauce for an authentic, delicious appetizer or side. Enjoy!

53. Vegetarian bibimbap

Ingredients:
- 1 cup short grain brown rice, cooked per package instructions
- 1 cup fresh spinach, blanched and drained
- 1/2 cup shredded carrots
- 1/2 cup bean sprouts
- 1/2 cup shitake mushrooms, sliced
- 1 cucumber, julienned
- 1 cup firm tofu, cubed and pan-fried until crispy
- 2 eggs (or just egg whites for vegetarian)
- 2 tablespoons gochujang (Korean chili paste)
- 2 tablespoons sesame oil
- 2 teaspoons sesame seeds
- 2 green onions, thinly sliced

Instructions:
1. Cook the brown rice according to package instructions. Set aside.

2. Prepare the vegetable toppings: blanch the spinach, shred the carrots, cook the bean sprouts briefly, sauté the mushrooms, julienne the cucumber, and pan-fry the tofu until crispy. Set aside.

3. In a stone bowl or skillet, create a bed of rice. Arrange the spinach, carrots, sprouts, mushrooms, cucumber and tofu over the rice in sections.

4. In a non-stick pan, fry the eggs sunny-side up, or cook the egg whites if avoiding eggs. Place in the center of the rice bowl.

5. In a small bowl, mix together the gochujang paste with 2-3 tablespoons of water to thin it out slightly.

6. Drizzle the sauced gochujang over the bibimbap in a spiral pattern.

7. Drizzle the sesame oil over everything and sprinkle with sesame seeds and green onions.

8. To eat, thoroughly mix all the ingredients together with a spoon, blending the flavors. The hot rice will lightly cook the raw vegetables.

This Korean rice dish is so flavorful with the mix of seasoned vegetables, crispy tofu, salty-sweet gochujang sauce and savory egg. Feel free to add any other veggies you enjoy like zucchini or steamed broccoli. Adjust the gochujang to taste for more or less heat and sauce.

54. Tofu lettuce wraps

Ingredients:
- 14 oz extra-firm tofu, drained and crumbled
- 2 tbsp olive oil
- 1 red bell pepper, diced
- 1 cup shredded carrots
- 4 green onions, sliced (separate white and green parts)
- 3 cloves garlic, minced
- 1 tbsp freshly grated ginger
- 2 tbsp low-sodium soy sauce
- 2 tsp rice vinegar
- 1 tsp sesame oil
- 1 tsp Sriracha or chili garlic sauce (optional)
- Salt and pepper to taste
- Butter or iceberg lettuce leaves
- Toppings: chopped cashews, fresh cilantro, lime wedges

Instructions:
1. Heat olive oil in a large skillet or wok over medium-high heat. Add the crumbled tofu and cook for 5 minutes until lightly browned, stirring occasionally.

2. Add the diced bell pepper, shredded carrots, white parts of the green onions, garlic and grated ginger. Stir-fry for 2-3 minutes.

3. Add the soy sauce, rice vinegar, sesame oil and Sriracha (if using). Toss everything to combine and cook for 2 more minutes.

4. Season with salt and pepper to taste. Remove from heat and stir in the green parts of the onions.

5. Scoop a few tablespoons of the tofu mixture into each lettuce leaf.

6. Top with cashews, fresh cilantro, and a squeeze of lime juice.

7. Serve the lettuce wraps immediately while the filling is warm.

These veggie-packed lettuce wraps make for such a fresh and flavorful light meal or appetizer. The tofu gets nice and crispy from browning first before adding the vegetables and sauce. The cashews give a nice crunch on top. Feel free to mix up the veggie varieties you use based on what you have on hand. Enjoy these low-carb, protein-packed lettuce wraps!

55. Mushroom and spinach frittata

Ingredients:
- 8 large eggs
- 1/4 cup milk or cream
- 1/2 tsp salt
- 1/4 tsp black pepper
- 2 tbsp olive oil
- 8 oz cremini or button mushrooms, sliced
- 1 shallot, diced
- 2 cloves garlic, minced
- 5 oz fresh baby spinach
- 1/2 cup shredded cheese (cheddar, Swiss, feta etc.)

Instructions:

1. Preheat oven to 375°F. Grease a 9-inch pie plate or oven-safe skillet with butter or non-stick spray.

2. In a medium bowl, whisk together the eggs, milk, salt and pepper until fully combined. Set aside.

3. Heat the olive oil in a skillet over medium-high heat. Add the sliced mushrooms and sauté for 5 minutes until starting to brown.

4. Add the diced shallot and garlic and cook for 2 more minutes until fragrant.

5. Add the spinach and continue cooking for 2-3 minutes until the spinach is wilted down.

6. Spread the mushroom and spinach mixture evenly into the prepared pie plate or skillet.

7. Pour the egg mixture over the veggies and sprinkle the shredded cheese evenly over the top.

8. Bake for 18-22 minutes until the eggs are completely set and the top is lightly golden brown.

9. Allow the frittata to cool for 5 minutes before slicing into wedges.

10. Serve the mushroom and spinach frittata warm garnished with extra black pepper, fresh herbs or a sprinkle of parmesan if desired.

This fluffy frittata packed with mushrooms, spinach and cheese makes a satisfying vegetarian breakfast, brunch or light dinner dish. The eggs puff up beautifully around the sauteed veggies. Feel free to use your favorite mushroom variety and cheese. You can also add other veggies like roasted red peppers or asparagus. Enjoy!

56. Grilled vegetable sandwiches with hummus

Ingredients:
- Assorted vegetables
- Olive oil
- Salt and pepper
- Bread slices
- Hummus
- Optional: tomatoes, avocado, lettuce, cheese

Instructions:

1. Preheat grill.

2. Slice and coat vegetables with oil, salt, and pepper.

3. Grill vegetables until tender.

4. Spread hummus on bread slices.

5. Layer grilled vegetables (and optional ingredients) between bread slices.

6. Optionally toast sandwich.

7. Slice and serve warm.

Enjoy your grilled vegetable sandwiches with hummus!

57. Spinach and ricotta stuffed shells

Ingredients:
- 20 jumbo pasta shells
- 2 cups ricotta cheese
- 1 cup chopped spinach (fresh or frozen, thawed and drained)
- 1 cup shredded mozzarella cheese
- 1/2 cup grated Parmesan cheese
- 1 egg
- 2 cloves garlic, minced
- 1 teaspoon dried basil
- 1 teaspoon dried oregano
- Salt and pepper to taste
- 2 cups marinara sauce

Instructions:
1. Preheat your oven to 350°F (175°C).

2. Cook the jumbo pasta shells according to package instructions until al dente. Drain and set aside to cool.

3. In a large mixing bowl, combine ricotta cheese, chopped spinach, mozzarella cheese, Parmesan cheese, egg, minced garlic, dried basil, dried oregano, salt, and pepper. Mix well until all ingredients are evenly incorporated.

4. Spread a thin layer of marinara sauce on the bottom of a baking dish.

5. Stuff each cooked pasta shell with the spinach and ricotta mixture, then place them in the baking dish.

6. Once all shells are stuffed and arranged in the baking dish, spoon the remaining marinara sauce over the top.

7. Sprinkle some extra mozzarella and Parmesan cheese on top of the shells.

8. Cover the baking dish with foil and bake in the preheated oven for 25-30 minutes, or until the cheese is melted and bubbly.

9. Remove the foil during the last 5 minutes of baking to allow the cheese to brown slightly.

10. Once done, remove from the oven and let it cool for a few minutes before serving. Serve warm and enjoy your delicious spinach and ricotta stuffed shells!

58. Baked ratatouille with cheese

Ingredients:
- 1 eggplant, sliced into rounds
- 2 zucchinis, sliced into rounds
- 2 bell peppers, sliced
- 2 tomatoes, sliced
- 1 onion, sliced
- 3 cloves garlic, minced
- 2 tablespoons olive oil
- Salt and pepper to taste
- 1 teaspoon dried thyme
- 1 teaspoon dried oregano
- 1/2 cup grated Parmesan cheese
- 1/2 cup shredded mozzarella cheese

Instructions:
1. Preheat your oven to 375°F (190°C).

2. Arrange the sliced eggplant, zucchini, bell peppers, tomatoes, onion, and minced garlic in overlapping layers in a baking dish.

3. Drizzle olive oil over the vegetables and season with salt, pepper, dried thyme, and dried oregano.

4. Cover the baking dish with aluminum foil and bake in the preheated oven for 30 minutes.
5. After 30 minutes, remove the foil and sprinkle the grated Parmesan cheese evenly over the top of the vegetables.

6. Return the baking dish to the oven and bake for an additional 15 minutes, or until the vegetables are tender and the cheese is melted and golden brown.

7. Once done, remove from the oven and sprinkle shredded mozzarella cheese over the top.

8. Return the baking dish to the oven and bake for another 5 minutes, or until the mozzarella cheese is melted and bubbly.

9. Remove from the oven and let it cool for a few minutes before serving. Serve warm and enjoy your delicious baked ratatouille with cheese!

This dish is versatile and can be served as a main course or a side dish. It's perfect for using up seasonal vegetables and is sure to be a hit with family and friends. Enjoy!

59. Chickpea salad with cucumber and tomatoes

Ingredients:
- 1 can (15 oz) chickpeas, drained and rinsed
- 1 cucumber, diced
- 2 cups cherry tomatoes, halved
- 1/4 red onion, finely chopped
- 1/4 cup fresh parsley, chopped
- 1/4 cup feta cheese, crumbled (optional)
- 3 tablespoons olive oil
- 1 tablespoon lemon juice
- 1 tablespoon red wine vinegar
- 1 clove garlic, minced
- Salt and pepper to taste

Instructions:
1. In a large bowl, combine chickpeas, cucumber, cherry tomatoes, red onion, and parsley.

2. In a small bowl, whisk together olive oil, lemon juice, red wine vinegar, minced garlic, salt, and pepper.

3. Pour the dressing over the chickpea mixture and toss to coat evenly.

4. If using, sprinkle crumbled feta cheese on top and gently mix.

5. Let the salad sit for at least 10 minutes to allow the flavors to meld.

6. Serve chilled or at room temperature.

Enjoy your refreshing chickpea salad with cucumber and tomatoes! This salad is perfect as a side dish or a light main course.

60. Vegetable biryani

Ingredients:
- 2 cups basmati rice, soaked
- 2 tbsp ghee or oil
- 1 large onion, sliced
- 2 tomatoes, chopped
- 1 cup mixed vegetables (carrots, peas, potatoes, cauliflower), diced
- 1/2 cup yogurt
- 1 tbsp ginger-garlic paste
- 2 green chilies, slit
- 1 tsp cumin seeds
- 1 tsp garam masala
- 1 tsp ground coriander
- 1/2 tsp turmeric
- 1/2 tsp red chili powder
- 1/4 tsp saffron strands (optional)
- 1/4 cup warm milk (if using saffron)
- Salt to taste
- Fresh cilantro for garnish
- Fried onions for garnish (optional)

Whole Spices:
- 2 bay leaves
- 4 green cardamom pods
- 4 cloves
- 1-inch cinnamon stick

Instructions:
1. Heat ghee/oil in a pot. Add whole spices and cumin seeds, sauté until fragrant.

2. Add onions, cook until golden. Add ginger-garlic paste and chilies, cook 1 minute.

3. Add tomatoes, cook until soft. Add vegetables, spices, and salt. Cook for a few minutes.

4. Stir in yogurt. Add drained rice, mix gently.

5. Add water to cover rice (about 3 1/2 cups). Bring to a boil, then simmer on low for 15-20 minutes.

6. If using saffron, soak in warm milk. Once rice is cooked, drizzle saffron milk over rice.

7. Garnish with cilantro and fried onions. Serve hot with raita.

61. Broccoli and cheddar quiche

Ingredients:
- 1 pie crust (store-bought or homemade)
- 2 cups broccoli florets, chopped
- 1 cup shredded cheddar cheese
- 4 large eggs
- 1 cup milk (whole milk or any milk of your choice)
- Salt and pepper to taste
- 1/4 teaspoon nutmeg (optional)
- 1/4 teaspoon garlic powder (optional)

Instructions:
1. Preheat your oven to 375°F (190°C).

2. Place the pie crust in a pie dish and crimp the edges. Prick the bottom of the crust with a fork to prevent bubbling.

3. Steam or blanch the broccoli florets until they are just tender, then drain and set aside.

4. Spread the shredded cheddar cheese evenly over the bottom of the pie crust.

5. Arrange the cooked broccoli florets on top of the cheese.

6. In a mixing bowl, whisk together the eggs, milk, salt, pepper, nutmeg (if using), and garlic powder (if using) until well combined.

7. Pour the egg mixture over the broccoli and cheese in the pie crust.

8. Place the quiche in the preheated oven and bake for 35-40 minutes, or until the center is set and the top is golden brown.

9. Once done, remove the quiche from the oven and let it cool for a few minutes before slicing.

10. Slice and serve warm or at room temperature.

Enjoy your delicious broccoli and cheddar quiche! It's perfect for breakfast, brunch, or a light dinner, and you can customize it with your favorite herbs and seasonings if desired.

62. Tofu tikka masala

Ingredients:
- 1 block (14 oz) firm tofu, pressed and cubed
- 1 onion, finely chopped
- 2 tomatoes, blended into a puree
- 1/2 cup plain yogurt (vegan yogurt for vegan option)
- 2 tablespoons tomato paste
- 2 cloves garlic, minced
- 1-inch ginger, grated
- 1 teaspoon ground cumin
- 1 teaspoon ground coriander
- 1 teaspoon paprika
- 1 teaspoon turmeric powder
- 1 teaspoon garam masala
- 1/2 teaspoon chili powder (adjust to taste)
- Salt to taste
- 2 tablespoons oil
- Fresh cilantro leaves for garnish
- Cooked rice or naan bread for serving

Instructions:
1. In a bowl, mix together yogurt, tomato paste, minced garlic, grated ginger, ground cumin, ground coriander, paprika, turmeric powder, garam masala, chili powder, and salt.

2. Add cubed tofu to the marinade, ensuring it's evenly coated. Let it marinate for at least 30 minutes or longer in the refrigerator.

3. Heat oil in a skillet over medium heat. Add finely chopped onions and sauté until golden brown.

4. Add the tofu along with the marinade to the skillet. Cook until the tofu is lightly browned on all sides.

5. Pour in the tomato puree and simmer for about 10-15 minutes until the sauce thickens and the flavors meld together.

6. Adjust seasoning according to taste preferences. Garnish with fresh cilantro leaves. Serve hot with cooked rice or naan bread.

Enjoy your flavorful tofu tikka masala! It's a satisfying and protein-packed vegetarian dish that's perfect for any occasion.

63. Roasted vegetable quinoa bowl

Ingredients:
- 1 cup quinoa, rinsed
- 2 cups water or vegetable broth
- Assorted vegetables (such as bell peppers, zucchini, cherry tomatoes, red onion, broccoli, carrots), chopped
- 2 tablespoons olive oil
- Salt and pepper to taste
- 1 teaspoon dried herbs (such as thyme, oregano, or rosemary)
- Optional additions: chickpeas, avocado, feta cheese, nuts or seeds
- **For the dressing:**
  - 3 tablespoons olive oil
  - 2 tablespoons balsamic vinegar
  - 1 tablespoon maple syrup or honey
  - 1 teaspoon Dijon mustard
  - Salt and pepper to taste

Instructions:
1. Preheat your oven to 400°F (200°C).

2. In a saucepan, combine quinoa and water or vegetable broth. Bring to a boil, then reduce heat, cover, and simmer for about 15-20 minutes, or until the quinoa is cooked and fluffy. Remove from heat and let it sit, covered, for 5 minutes. Fluff with a fork.

3. While the quinoa is cooking, spread chopped vegetables on a baking sheet. Drizzle with olive oil, season with salt, pepper, and dried herbs, and toss to coat evenly.

4. Roast the vegetables in the preheated oven for about 20-25 minutes, or until they are tender and lightly browned, stirring halfway through.

5. In a small bowl, whisk together olive oil, balsamic vinegar, maple syrup or honey, Dijon mustard, salt, and pepper to make the dressing.

6. To assemble the bowls, divide cooked quinoa among serving bowls. Top with roasted vegetables and any optional additions like chickpeas, avocado, feta cheese, nuts, or seeds.

7. Drizzle the dressing over the bowls or serve it on the side. Serve the roasted vegetable quinoa bowls warm and enjoy!

These bowls are versatile, customizable, and perfect for a healthy lunch or dinner. Feel free to mix and match vegetables and toppings according to your preference.

64. Spinach and goat cheese pizza on whole wheat crust

Ingredients:
- 1 whole wheat pizza crust (store-bought or homemade)
- 2 cups fresh spinach leaves, washed and dried
- 4 oz goat cheese, crumbled
- 1/4 cup shredded mozzarella cheese
- 2 cloves garlic, minced
- 1 tablespoon olive oil
- Salt and pepper to taste
- Red pepper flakes (optional)
- Cornmeal or flour for dusting

Instructions:

1. Preheat your oven to the temperature specified on the pizza crust package or to 425°F (220°C).

2. If using homemade pizza dough, roll it out on a floured surface into your desired shape and thickness. Transfer the dough to a pizza stone or baking sheet sprinkled with cornmeal or flour.

3. In a skillet, heat olive oil over medium heat. Add minced garlic and sauté for about 1 minute until fragrant.

4. Add fresh spinach leaves to the skillet and sauté until wilted, about 2-3 minutes. Season with salt, pepper, and red pepper flakes if desired. Remove from heat.

5. Spread the wilted spinach evenly over the prepared pizza crust.

6. Sprinkle crumbled goat cheese and shredded mozzarella cheese over the spinach.

7. Bake the pizza in the preheated oven for 12-15 minutes, or until the crust is golden brown and the cheese is melted and bubbly.

8. Once done, remove the pizza from the oven and let it cool for a few minutes before slicing. Slice the spinach and goat cheese pizza into wedges and serve hot.

Enjoy your delicious and wholesome spinach and goat cheese pizza on whole wheat crust! It's a flavorful and nutritious meal that's perfect for a quick dinner or weekend treat.

65. Stuffed grape leaves with rice and herbs

Ingredients:
- Grape leaves (jarred)
- 1 cup short-grain rice
- Herbs: parsley, dill, mint
- Olive oil
- Onion, garlic
- Lemon juice
- Salt, pepper
- Water or vegetable broth

Instructions:

1. Mix rice, herbs, toasted pine nuts (optional), sautéed onion, garlic, lemon juice, salt, and pepper.

2. Fill grape leaves with mixture, roll tightly.

3. Place in pot, cover with water or broth, simmer 30-40 mins.

4. Serve warm or at room temperature.

Enjoy your stuffed grape leaves with rice and herbs!

66. Vegetarian pad Thai

Ingredients:
- 8 oz rice noodles
- 2 tablespoons oil (vegetable or peanut)
- 2 cloves garlic, minced
- 1 block (14 oz) firm tofu, pressed and cubed
- 2 cups mixed vegetables (such as bell
  peppers, carrots, broccoli, snap peas)
- 3 green onions, sliced
- 2 eggs, lightly beaten (omit for vegan option)
- 1/4 cup chopped peanuts
- Lime wedges for serving
- Fresh cilantro for garnish

For the sauce:
- 3 tablespoons soy sauce
- 2 tablespoons brown sugar
- 1 tablespoon rice vinegar
- 1 tablespoon lime juice
- 1 tablespoon tamarind
paste or substitute with
additional lime juice
- 1 teaspoon sriracha or chili
sauce (adjust to taste)

Instructions:

1. Cook rice noodles according to package instructions until al dente. Drain and set aside.

2. In a small bowl, whisk together the sauce ingredients: soy sauce, brown sugar, rice vinegar, lime juice, tamarind paste, and sriracha. Set aside.

3. Heat oil in a large skillet or wok over medium-high heat. Add minced garlic and cubed tofu. Cook until tofu is golden brown on all sides.

4. Add mixed vegetables and sliced green onions to the skillet. Stir-fry for a few minutes until vegetables are tender-crisp.

5. Push tofu and vegetables to one side of the skillet. Pour beaten eggs into the empty side and scramble until cooked.

6. Add cooked rice noodles and prepared sauce to the skillet. Toss everything together until well combined and heated through.

7. Remove from heat and sprinkle chopped peanuts on top.

8. Serve vegetarian Pad Thai hot, garnished with lime wedges and fresh cilantro.

Enjoy your flavorful vegetarian Pad Thai! It's a delicious and versatile dish that's perfect for a quick and satisfying meal.

67. Lentil and vegetable soup

Ingredients:
- 1 cup dried lentils, rinsed and drained
- 1 onion, chopped
- 2 carrots, diced
- 2 celery stalks, diced
- 2 cloves garlic, minced
- 1 can (14 oz) diced tomatoes
- 6 cups vegetable broth
- 1 teaspoon dried thyme
- 1 teaspoon dried oregano
- 1 bay leaf
- Salt and pepper to taste
- 2 tablespoons olive oil
- Fresh parsley for garnish (optional)

Instructions:
1. Heat olive oil in a large pot over medium heat. Add chopped onion, carrots, and celery. Sauté until vegetables are softened, about 5 minutes.

2. Add minced garlic and sauté for another minute until fragrant.

3. Stir in dried lentils, diced tomatoes, vegetable broth, dried thyme, dried oregano, bay leaf, salt, and pepper.

4. Bring the soup to a boil, then reduce the heat to low. Cover and simmer for about 25-30 minutes, or until the lentils and vegetables are tender.

5. Once the soup is done cooking, taste and adjust seasoning if needed.

6. Remove the bay leaf from the soup.

7. Serve the lentil and vegetable soup hot, garnished with fresh parsley if desired.

Enjoy your hearty and flavorful lentil and vegetable soup! It's perfect for a comforting meal, especially on chilly days.

68. Caprese stuffed avocados

Ingredients:
- 2 ripe avocados
- 1 cup cherry tomatoes, halved
- 1 cup fresh mozzarella balls (or diced fresh mozzarella)
- Fresh basil leaves, torn
- Balsamic glaze or balsamic reduction, for drizzling
- Extra virgin olive oil, for drizzling
- Salt and pepper to taste

Instructions:

1. Cut the avocados in half lengthwise and remove the pits.

2. Scoop out a little flesh from each avocado half to create a larger cavity for the filling.

3. In a bowl, combine cherry tomatoes, fresh mozzarella balls, and torn basil leaves.

4. Season the mixture with salt and pepper to taste.

5. Fill each avocado half with the caprese mixture, pressing gently to pack it in.

6. Drizzle the stuffed avocados with balsamic glaze or balsamic reduction, and extra virgin olive oil.

7. Optionally, sprinkle with additional salt and pepper to taste.

8. Serve immediately as a tasty appetizer or light meal.

Enjoy your delicious and fresh Caprese stuffed avocados! They're perfect for a quick and healthy snack or as part of a summer meal.

69. Butternut squash risotto

Ingredients:
- 1 small butternut squash, peeled, seeded, and diced
- 4 cups vegetable broth
- 2 tablespoons olive oil
- 1 small onion, finely chopped
- 2 cloves garlic, minced
- 1 1/2 cups Arborio rice
- 1/2 cup dry white wine (optional)
- 1/2 cup grated Parmesan cheese (plus extra for serving)
- Salt and pepper to taste
- Fresh parsley or sage leaves for garnish (optional)

Instructions:
1. In a saucepan, bring the vegetable broth to a simmer. Keep it warm over low heat.

2. Heat olive oil in a large skillet or pot over medium heat. Add chopped onion and cook until softened, about 5 minutes.

3. Add minced garlic and diced butternut squash to the skillet. Cook for another 5 minutes, stirring occasionally.

4. Stir in Arborio rice and cook for 1-2 minutes until the rice is coated with oil and lightly toasted.

5. If using, pour in the white wine and cook until it's mostly absorbed by the rice.

6. Begin adding the warm vegetable broth to the skillet, one ladleful at a time, stirring frequently. Wait until each addition of broth is mostly absorbed before adding more.

7. Continue adding broth and stirring until the rice is creamy and tender, about 20-25 minutes in total.

8. Once the rice is cooked to your desired consistency, stir in grated Parmesan cheese until melted and well combined.

9. Season the risotto with salt and pepper to taste. Remove the risotto from heat and let it rest for a couple of minutes. Serve the butternut squash risotto hot, garnished with additional grated Parmesan cheese and fresh parsley or sage leaves if desired.

70. Vegetable pot pie with whole wheat crust

Ingredients:
For the filling:
- 2 tbsp olive oil
- 1 onion, diced
- 2 cloves garlic, minced
- 2 carrots, diced
- 2 stalks celery, diced
- 1 cup mushrooms, sliced
- 1 cup frozen peas
- 1 cup frozen corn kernels
- 1 tsp dried thyme
- 1/2 tsp dried rosemary
- Salt and pepper to taste
- 3 tbsp all-purpose flour
- 2 cups vegetable broth
- 1/2 cup unsweetened almond milk
- 1 tbsp soy sauce or tamari

For the whole wheat crust:
- 1 1/2 cups whole wheat flour
- 1/2 tsp salt
- 1/2 cup vegan butter or coconut oil
- 4-6 tbsp ice water

Instructions:

1. Sauté onion, garlic, carrots, celery, and mushrooms. Add peas, corn, thyme, rosemary, salt, pepper, and flour. Pour in broth, almond milk, and soy sauce. Simmer until thickened.

2. Make the crust by mixing flour, salt, and vegan butter. Gradually add ice water until dough forms. Roll out half for the bottom crust, and the other half for the top.

3. Fill a pie dish with the vegetable filling. Cover with the top crust, seal edges, and cut slits on top. Bake at 375°F (190°C) for 40-45 minutes until golden brown.

Enjoy your veggie pot pie with a wholesome whole wheat crust!

71. Baked spinach and cheese stuffed tomatoes

Ingredients:
- 4 large tomatoes
- 2 cups fresh spinach, chopped
- 1 clove garlic, minced
- 1/2 cup shredded vegan cheese (such as vegan mozzarella or cheddar)
- 2 tablespoons nutritional yeast (optional)
- Salt and pepper to taste
- Olive oil, for drizzling
- Fresh basil leaves, for garnish (optional)

Instructions:
1. Preheat your oven to 375°F (190°C). Line a baking dish with parchment paper or lightly grease it with olive oil.

2. Slice off the tops of the tomatoes and carefully scoop out the seeds and pulp with a spoon, leaving the tomato shells intact. Set aside.

3. In a skillet, heat a drizzle of olive oil over medium heat. Add the minced garlic and chopped spinach. Sauté until the spinach is wilted and the garlic is fragrant, about 2-3 minutes. Remove from heat.

4. In a mixing bowl, combine the sautéed spinach and garlic with the shredded vegan cheese and nutritional yeast (if using). Season with salt and pepper to taste.

5. Stuff each hollowed-out tomato with the spinach and cheese mixture, pressing down gently to pack it in.

6. Place the stuffed tomatoes in the prepared baking dish. Drizzle with a little olive oil and sprinkle with additional salt and pepper if desired.

7. Bake in the preheated oven for 20-25 minutes, or until the tomatoes are tender and the filling is hot and bubbly.

8. Remove from the oven and let the stuffed tomatoes cool for a few minutes before serving.

9. Garnish with fresh basil leaves if desired.

Enjoy your delicious baked spinach and cheese stuffed tomatoes as a flavorful appetizer or side dish!

72. Tofu and vegetable stir-fry noodles

Ingredients:
- 8 oz (225g) rice noodles or any noodles of your choice
- 1 block (14 oz/400g) firm tofu, drained and cubed
- 2 tablespoons soy sauce or tamari
- 2 tablespoons vegetable oil
- 2 cloves garlic, minced
- 1 tablespoon grated ginger
- 1 onion, thinly sliced
- 1 bell pepper, thinly sliced
- 1 carrot, julienned
- 1 cup broccoli florets
- 1 cup snap peas, trimmed
- 2 tablespoons hoisin sauce
- 2 tablespoons rice vinegar
- 1 tablespoon sesame oil
- Sesame seeds and chopped green onions for garnish (optional)

Instructions:
1. Cook the noodles according to the package instructions. Drain and set aside.

2. In a bowl, marinate the tofu cubes with soy sauce or tamari for about 10-15 minutes.

3. Heat 1 tablespoon of vegetable oil in a large skillet or wok over medium-high heat. Add the marinated tofu cubes and cook until golden brown and crispy on all sides, about 5-7 minutes. Remove the tofu from the skillet and set aside.

4. In the same skillet, heat the remaining tablespoon of vegetable oil over medium heat. Add the minced garlic and grated ginger, and cook for about 1 minute until fragrant.

5. Add the sliced onion, bell pepper, julienned carrot, broccoli florets, and snap peas to the skillet. Stir-fry for about 5-7 minutes until the vegetables are tender-crisp.

6. Return the cooked tofu to the skillet. Add the cooked noodles, hoisin sauce, rice vinegar, and sesame oil. Toss everything together until well combined and heated through.

7. Taste and adjust seasoning if needed, adding more soy sauce or tamari if desired. Serve the tofu and vegetable stir-fry noodles hot, garnished with sesame seeds and chopped green onions if desired.

Enjoy your delicious tofu and vegetable stir-fry noodles as a satisfying and flavorful meal!

73. Stuffed bell peppers with lentils and rice

Ingredients:
- 4 large bell peppers (any color)
- 1 cup cooked brown rice
- 1 cup cooked lentils (green or brown)
- 1 tablespoon olive oil
- 1 onion, diced
- 2 cloves garlic, minced
- 1 carrot, diced
- 1 stalk celery, diced
- 1 cup diced tomatoes (fresh or canned)
- 1 teaspoon dried oregano
- 1 teaspoon dried basil
- Salt and pepper to taste
- 1/2 cup shredded vegan cheese (optional)
- Fresh parsley, chopped (for garnish)

Instructions:

1. Preheat your oven to 375°F (190°C). Prepare a baking dish by lightly greasing it with olive oil or lining it with parchment paper.

2. Cut the tops off the bell peppers and remove the seeds and membranes from the inside. If necessary, slice a small portion from the bottom of each pepper to help them stand upright. Place the peppers in the prepared baking dish and set aside.

3. In a large skillet, heat the olive oil over medium heat. Add the diced onion, minced garlic, diced carrot, and diced celery. Sauté for 5-7 minutes until the vegetables are softened.

4. Add the cooked brown rice, cooked lentils, diced tomatoes, dried oregano, and dried basil to the skillet. Season with salt and pepper to taste. Stir to combine and cook for another 2-3 minutes until heated through.

5. Spoon the lentil and rice mixture into each bell pepper until they are filled to the top. If desired, sprinkle shredded vegan cheese on top of each stuffed pepper.

6. Cover the baking dish with aluminum foil and bake in the preheated oven for 25-30 minutes, or until the peppers are tender.

7. Remove the foil and bake for an additional 5-10 minutes, or until the cheese is melted and bubbly (if using).

8. Remove from the oven and let the stuffed bell peppers cool for a few minutes before serving. Garnish with chopped fresh parsley before serving, if desired.

74. Mushroom and spinach stuffed shells

Ingredients:
- 20 jumbo pasta shells
- 2 tablespoons olive oil
- 1 onion, diced
- 3 cloves garlic, minced
- 8 oz (225g) mushrooms, finely chopped
- 4 cups fresh spinach leaves
- 1 cup ricotta cheese (or vegan ricotta)
- 1/2 cup shredded mozzarella cheese (or vegan mozzarella)
- 1/4 cup grated Parmesan cheese (or vegan Parmesan)
- 1 teaspoon dried oregano
- Salt and pepper to taste
- 2 cups marinara sauce
- Fresh parsley, chopped, for garnish (optional)

Instructions:

1. Preheat your oven to 375°F (190°C). Grease a baking dish with olive oil or cooking spray.

2. Cook the jumbo pasta shells according to the package instructions until al dente. Drain and set aside.

3. In a large skillet, heat the olive oil over medium heat. Add the diced onion and minced garlic, and cook until softened and fragrant, about 3-4 minutes.

4. Add the chopped mushrooms to the skillet and cook until they release their moisture and start to brown, about 5-7 minutes.

5. Add the fresh spinach leaves to the skillet and cook until wilted, about 2-3 minutes. Remove from heat and let the mixture cool slightly.

6. In a mixing bowl, combine the ricotta cheese, shredded mozzarella cheese, grated Parmesan cheese, dried oregano, salt, and pepper. Add the cooked mushroom and spinach mixture to the bowl and mix until well combined.

7. Spoon the cheese and vegetable mixture into each cooked pasta shell, filling them to the brim. Spread a thin layer of marinara sauce on the bottom of the prepared baking dish. Arrange the stuffed shells in the dish in a single layer.

8. Pour the remaining marinara sauce over the stuffed shells, covering them evenly. Cover the baking dish with aluminum foil and bake in the preheated oven for 25-30 minutes, or until the shells are heated through and the sauce is bubbly.

9. Remove the foil and bake for an additional 5-10 minutes, or until the cheese is melted and golden brown. Remove from the oven and let the mushroom and spinach stuffed shells cool for a few minutes before serving. Garnish with chopped fresh parsley before serving, if desired.

75. Vegetable birria tacos

Ingredients:

For the birria sauce:
- 2 dried guajillo chilies
- 2 dried ancho chilies
- 1 onion, chopped
- 4 cloves garlic, minced
- 1 tablespoon ground cumin
- 1 tablespoon dried oregano
- 1 teaspoon smoked paprika
- 1 teaspoon ground cinnamon
- 1/2 teaspoon ground cloves
- 1/2 teaspoon ground coriander
- 4 cups vegetable broth
- 1 tablespoon vegetable oil
- Salt and pepper to taste

For the tacos:
- 8 small corn tortillas
- 2 cups mixed vegetables (such as bell peppers, onions, zucchini, mushrooms), sliced
- 1 tablespoon vegetable oil
- Chopped fresh cilantro, for garnish
- Lime wedges, for serving

Instructions:

1. Prepare the birria sauce: Remove the stems and seeds from the dried guajillo and ancho chilies. Place them in a bowl and cover with hot water. Let them soak for about 15-20 minutes until softened.

2. In a blender, combine the soaked chilies (drained), chopped onion, minced garlic, ground cumin, dried oregano, smoked paprika, ground cinnamon, ground cloves, ground coriander, and vegetable broth. Blend until smooth.

3. Heat the vegetable oil in a large pot over medium heat. Pour the blended sauce into the pot and bring to a simmer. Cook for about 15-20 minutes, stirring occasionally, until the sauce thickens. Season with salt and pepper to taste.

4. While the sauce is simmering, prepare the mixed vegetables for the tacos. Heat the vegetable oil in a skillet over medium-high heat. Add the sliced vegetables and sauté for 5-7 minutes until they are tender-crisp.

5. Warm the corn tortillas in a dry skillet or on a comal until they are soft and pliable.

6. To assemble the tacos, dip each tortilla into the simmering birria sauce to coat it lightly. Place a spoonful of sautéed mixed vegetables in the center of each tortilla. Fold the tortillas in half to form tacos.

7. Serve the vegetable birria tacos hot, garnished with chopped fresh cilantro and lime wedges on the side.

76. Lentil moussaka

Ingredients:
For the lentil filling:
- 1 cup dry lentils
- 3 cups vegetable broth
- 1 tbsp olive oil
- 1 onion, diced
- 2 cloves garlic, minced
- Assorted diced vegetables
(carrot, celery, bell pepper, zucchini)
- 1 can diced tomatoes
- 2 tbsp tomato paste
- Spices: oregano, thyme, cumin, salt, and pepper

For the potato and eggplant layers:
- 2 large potatoes, thinly sliced
- 1 large eggplant, thinly sliced
- Olive oil, salt, and pepper

For the béchamel sauce:
- 2 tbsp vegan butter or olive oil
- 3 tbsp all-purpose flour
- 2 cups unsweetened almond milk
- Spices: nutmeg, salt, and pepper
- 1/4 cup nutritional yeast (optional)

Instructions:
1. Cook lentils in vegetable broth until tender, then set aside.

2. Sauté onion, garlic, and assorted vegetables until softened.

3. Add diced tomatoes, tomato paste, and spices to the vegetable mixture. Cook until thickened.

4. Arrange sliced potatoes and eggplant on a baking sheet. Brush with olive oil, salt, and pepper. Bake until tender.

5. Prepare the béchamel sauce by melting vegan butter, whisking in flour, then gradually adding almond milk. Season with nutmeg, salt, and pepper.

6. Assemble moussaka layers: lentil filling, baked potato, eggplant, repeat.

7. Pour béchamel sauce over the top layer.

8. Bake until golden brown and bubbly. Let cool slightly before serving.

77. Quinoa stuffed eggplant

Ingredients:
- 2 large eggplants
- 1 cup quinoa, rinsed
- 2 cups vegetable broth or water
- 2 tbsp olive oil
- 1 onion, diced
- 2 cloves garlic, minced
- Assorted diced vegetables (bell pepper, zucchini, tomato)
- Fresh parsley and basil
- 1 tsp dried oregano
- Salt and pepper
- 1/4 cup grated Parmesan cheese or nutritional yeast (optional)
- Lemon wedges, for serving

Instructions:
1. Preheat oven to 400°F (200°C). Cut eggplants in half, score flesh, drizzle with oil, salt, and pepper, then roast for 25-30 min.

2. Cook quinoa in vegetable broth until tender.

3. Sauté onion and garlic, then add diced vegetables and cook until tender. Stir in cooked quinoa, herbs, and seasoning.

4. Scoop out eggplant flesh to create a hollow, then fill each half with quinoa mixture.

5. Bake stuffed eggplants for 10-15 min until heated through.

6. Serve with lemon wedges.

Enjoy your tasty quinoa stuffed eggplants!

78. Vegetable korma

Ingredients:
- 2 tablespoons vegetable oil
- 1 onion, finely chopped
- 2 cloves garlic, minced
- 1-inch piece of ginger, grated
- 2 green chilies, finely chopped (optional)
- 2 carrots, diced
- 1 potato, diced
- 1 cup cauliflower florets
- 1 cup green beans, cut into 1-inch pieces
- 1 cup peas (fresh or frozen)
- 1/2 cup cashews, soaked in water for 30 minutes
- 1 cup coconut milk
- 1 teaspoon ground turmeric
- 1 teaspoon ground cumin
- 1 teaspoon ground coriander
- 1/2 teaspoon garam masala
- Salt to taste
- Fresh cilantro leaves, for garnish

Instructions:

1. Heat the vegetable oil in a large skillet or pot over medium heat. Add the chopped onion and sauté until soft and translucent, about 5 minutes.

2. Add the minced garlic, grated ginger, and chopped green chilies (if using). Sauté for another 2 minutes until fragrant.

3. Add the diced carrots, potato, cauliflower florets, and green beans to the skillet. Cook for 5-7 minutes until the vegetables start to soften.

4. Drain the soaked cashews and transfer them to a blender. Add 1/2 cup of water and blend until smooth to make cashew cream.

5. Pour the cashew cream into the skillet with the vegetables. Stir in the coconut milk, ground turmeric, ground cumin, ground coriander, garam masala, and salt to taste. Mix well to combine.

6. Bring the mixture to a simmer, then reduce the heat to low. Cover and cook for 15-20 minutes, stirring occasionally, until the vegetables are tender and the sauce has thickened.

7. Stir in the peas and cook for another 2-3 minutes until heated through.

8. Taste and adjust seasoning if necessary. Serve the vegetable korma hot, garnished with fresh cilantro leaves.

79. Tofu and vegetable curry

Ingredients:
- 14 oz (400g) firm tofu, drained and cubed
- 2 tablespoons vegetable oil
- 1 onion, diced
- 2 cloves garlic, minced
- 1 tablespoon grated ginger
- 2 tablespoons curry powder
- 1 teaspoon ground turmeric
- 1 teaspoon ground cumin
- 1 teaspoon ground coriander
- 1 can (14 oz/400ml) coconut milk
- 1 cup vegetable broth
- 2 cups mixed vegetables (such as bell peppers, carrots, broccoli, peas)
- Salt and pepper to taste
- Fresh cilantro leaves, for garnish (optional)

Instructions:
1. Heat the vegetable oil in a large skillet or pot over medium heat. Add the diced onion and sauté until soft and translucent, about 5 minutes.

2. Add the minced garlic and grated ginger to the skillet. Sauté for another 2 minutes until fragrant.

3. Stir in the curry powder, ground turmeric, ground cumin, and ground coriander. Cook for 1-2 minutes to toast the spices.

4. Add the cubed tofu to the skillet and cook for 5 minutes, stirring occasionally, until lightly browned on all sides.

5. Pour in the coconut milk and vegetable broth. Stir to combine and bring the mixture to a simmer.

6. Add the mixed vegetables to the skillet. Cover and simmer for 10-15 minutes, or until the vegetables are tender.

7. Season the curry with salt and pepper to taste. Serve the tofu and vegetable curry hot, garnished with fresh cilantro leaves if desired.

Enjoy your flavorful tofu and vegetable curry served with rice or naan!

80. Stuffed poblano peppers with black beans and corn

Ingredients:
- 4 large poblano peppers
- 1 cup cooked black beans
- 1 cup corn kernels (fresh, canned, or frozen)
- 1 small onion, diced
- 2 cloves garlic, minced
- 1 teaspoon ground cumin
- 1 teaspoon chili powder
- 1/2 teaspoon smoked paprika
- Salt and pepper to taste
- 1 cup cooked rice (white or brown)
- 1 cup shredded cheese (cheddar, Monterey Jack, or vegan cheese)
- Fresh cilantro leaves, chopped, for garnish (optional)
- Lime wedges, for serving

Instructions:
1. Preheat your oven to 400°F (200°C). Line a baking sheet with parchment paper.

2. Cut a slit lengthwise down the center of each poblano pepper, leaving the stems intact. Carefully remove the seeds and membranes from the inside of the peppers.

3. In a skillet, heat a drizzle of oil over medium heat. Add the diced onion and minced garlic, and sauté until softened, about 3-4 minutes.

4. Add the cooked black beans, corn kernels, ground cumin, chili powder, smoked paprika, salt, and pepper to the skillet. Stir to combine and cook for another 2-3 minutes until heated through.

5. Remove the skillet from heat and stir in the cooked rice and half of the shredded cheese until well combined.

6. Stuff each poblano pepper with the black bean and corn mixture, pressing down gently to pack it in. Place the stuffed peppers on the prepared baking sheet.

7. Sprinkle the remaining shredded cheese over the top of each stuffed pepper.

8. Bake in the preheated oven for 20-25 minutes, or until the peppers are tender and the cheese is melted and bubbly.

9. Remove from the oven and let the stuffed poblano peppers cool for a few minutes before serving. Garnish with chopped fresh cilantro leaves and serve with lime wedges on the side.

81. Vegetarian bibimbap bowl

Ingredients:
For the bibimbap sauce:
- 1/4 cup soy sauce
- 2 tablespoons sesame oil
- 1 tablespoon honey or brown sugar
- 1 tablespoon rice vinegar
- 2 cloves garlic, minced
- 1 teaspoon grated ginger
- 1 teaspoon gochujang (Korean chili paste) (optional)

For the bibimbap bowl:
- 2 cups cooked rice (white or brown)
- 1 cup sliced mixed vegetables (such as carrots, zucchini, bell peppers, mushrooms, spinach)
- 1 cup bean sprouts, blanched
- 1 cup shredded lettuce or baby spinach
- 4 fried or poached eggs (omit for vegan option)
- Toasted sesame seeds, for garnish
- Sliced green onions, for garnish
- Kimchi, for serving (optional)

Instructions:
1. In a small bowl, whisk together the soy sauce, sesame oil, honey or brown sugar, rice vinegar, minced garlic, grated ginger, and gochujang (if using) to make the bibimbap sauce. Set aside.

2. Divide the cooked rice among serving bowls.

3. In a large skillet or wok, stir-fry the sliced mixed vegetables over medium-high heat until they are tender-crisp, about 5-7 minutes.

4. Divide the stir-fried vegetables, blanched bean sprouts, and shredded lettuce or baby spinach among the serving bowls on top of the rice.

5. If using, fry or poach eggs and place one on top of each bowl.

6. Drizzle the bibimbap sauce over the bowls and garnish with toasted sesame seeds and sliced green onions.

7. Serve the vegetarian bibimbap bowls immediately with kimchi on the side if desired.

82. Lentil and vegetable shepherd's pie

Ingredients:
For the lentil filling:
- 1 cup dry lentils
- 3 cups vegetable broth
- 2 tbsp olive oil
- 1 onion, diced
- 2 cloves garlic, minced
- Assorted diced vegetables (carrots, celery, bell pepper, mushrooms)
- Spices: thyme, rosemary, paprika, salt, pepper
- 2 tbsp tomato paste
- 1 tbsp soy sauce
- 1 cup frozen peas

For the mashed potato topping:
- 4 large potatoes, peeled and chopped
- 1/4 cup unsweetened almond milk
- 2 tbsp vegan butter
- Salt and pepper

Instructions:

1. Cook lentils in vegetable broth until tender, then set aside.

2. Boil potatoes until tender, then mash with almond milk, vegan butter, salt, and pepper.

3. Sauté onion and garlic, then add diced vegetables and cook until tender. Stir in cooked lentils, tomato paste, soy sauce, and peas.

4. Transfer lentil mixture to a baking dish, top with mashed potatoes, and bake until golden brown.

5. Let cool slightly before serving.

Enjoy your lentil and vegetable shepherd's pie!

83. Stuffed portobello mushrooms with quinoa and cheese

Ingredients:
For the lentil filling:
- 1 cup dry lentils
- 3 cups vegetable broth
- 2 tbsp olive oil
- 1 onion, diced
- 2 cloves garlic, minced
- Assorted diced vegetables (carrots, celery, bell pepper, mushrooms)
- Spices: thyme, rosemary, paprika, salt, pepper
- 2 tbsp tomato paste
- 1 tbsp soy sauce
- 1 cup frozen peas

For the mashed potato topping:
- 4 large potatoes, peeled and chopped
- 1/4 cup unsweetened almond milk
- 2 tbsp vegan butter
- Salt and pepper

Instructions:

1. Cook lentils until tender in vegetable broth. Drain and set aside.

2. Boil potatoes until tender, then mash with almond milk, vegan butter, salt, and pepper.

3. Sauté onion and garlic, then add diced vegetables and cook until tender.

4. Add spices, cooked lentils, tomato paste, and soy sauce to the skillet. Stir in frozen peas.

5. Transfer lentil mixture to a baking dish and spread mashed potatoes on top.

6. Bake until heated through and potatoes are golden brown.

7. Let cool slightly before serving.

Enjoy your lentil and vegetable shepherd's pie!

84. Vegetable and tofu spring rolls

Ingredients:
For the spring rolls:
- 8 rice paper wrappers
- 1 block firm tofu, sliced into thin strips
- 1 carrot, julienned
- 1 cucumber, julienned
- 1 bell pepper, thinly sliced
- 1 cup shredded lettuce or cabbage
- 1/2 cup fresh mint leaves
- 1/2 cup fresh cilantro leaves
- 1/4 cup chopped peanuts or cashews (optional)
- Lime wedges, for serving (optional)

For the dipping sauce:
- 1/4 cup soy sauce or tamari
- 2 tablespoons rice vinegar
- 1 tablespoon honey or maple syrup
- 1 teaspoon sesame oil
- 1 clove garlic, minced
- 1 teaspoon grated ginger
- Red pepper flakes, to taste (optional)

Instructions:

1. Prepare the tofu: Heat a skillet over medium heat and lightly oil it. Cook tofu slices until golden brown and crispy on both sides, about 3-4 minutes per side. Set aside.

2. Fill a large shallow dish with warm water. Dip one rice paper wrapper into the water for a few seconds until it becomes pliable. Remove and place it on a clean work surface.

3. Arrange a few strips of tofu, julienned carrot, cucumber, bell pepper, shredded lettuce or cabbage, mint leaves, and cilantro leaves in the center of the wrapper.

4. Sprinkle with chopped peanuts or cashews if desired.

5. Fold the bottom edge of the wrapper over the filling, then fold in the sides, and roll up tightly.

6. Repeat with the remaining wrappers and filling ingredients.

7. In a small bowl, whisk together all ingredients for the dipping sauce until well combined.

8. Serve the spring rolls with the dipping sauce and lime wedges on the side.

Enjoy your delicious vegetable and tofu spring rolls as a light and refreshing appetizer or snack!

85. Chickpea and vegetable tagine

Ingredients:
- 2 tablespoons olive oil
- 1 onion, diced
- 2 cloves garlic, minced
- 1 teaspoon ground cumin
- 1 teaspoon ground coriander
- 1 teaspoon ground cinnamon
- 1/2 teaspoon ground turmeric
- 1/4 teaspoon cayenne pepper (optional, for heat)
- 1 can (14 oz/400g) chickpeas, drained and rinsed
- 1 can (14 oz/400g) diced tomatoes
- 1 cup vegetable broth
- 1 sweet potato, peeled and diced
- 2 carrots, peeled and sliced
- 1 zucchini, diced
- 1 red bell pepper, diced
- 1/2 cup dried apricots, chopped
- Salt and pepper to taste
- Fresh cilantro leaves, chopped, for garnish (optional)
- Cooked couscous or rice, for serving

Instructions:
1. Heat the olive oil in a large skillet or Dutch oven over medium heat. Add the diced onion and sauté until softened, about 5 minutes.

2. Add the minced garlic, ground cumin, ground coriander, ground cinnamon, ground turmeric, and cayenne pepper (if using). Cook for another 1-2 minutes until fragrant.

3. Stir in the drained chickpeas, diced tomatoes, vegetable broth, diced sweet potato, sliced carrots, diced zucchini, diced red bell pepper, and chopped dried apricots.

4. Season with salt and pepper to taste. Stir well to combine.

5. Bring the mixture to a simmer, then reduce the heat to low. Cover and cook for 20-25 minutes, stirring occasionally, until the vegetables are tender and the flavors have melded together.

6. Taste and adjust seasoning if necessary. Serve the chickpea and vegetable tagine hot, garnished with chopped fresh cilantro leaves if desired. Serve over cooked couscous or rice

86. Spinach and cheese stuffed zucchini

Ingredients:
- 4 medium zucchinis
- 2 tablespoons olive oil
- 1 small onion, finely chopped
- 2 cloves garlic, minced
- 4 cups fresh spinach, chopped
- 1/2 cup ricotta cheese
- 1/2 cup grated Parmesan cheese
- 1/2 cup shredded mozzarella cheese
- Salt and pepper to taste
- Fresh basil leaves, chopped, for garnish (optional)

Instructions:
1. Preheat your oven to 375°F (190°C). Grease a baking dish with olive oil or cooking spray.

2. Cut the zucchinis in half lengthwise. Use a spoon to scoop out the flesh from the center of each zucchini half, leaving about 1/4 inch border around the edges. Chop the scooped out flesh and set aside.

3. In a large skillet, heat the olive oil over medium heat. Add the chopped onion and minced garlic, and sauté until softened, about 3-4 minutes.

4. Add the chopped spinach to the skillet and cook until wilted, about 2-3 minutes.

5. Stir in the chopped zucchini flesh and cook for another 2-3 minutes.

6. Remove the skillet from heat and transfer the mixture to a large mixing bowl.

7. Add the ricotta cheese, grated Parmesan cheese, and shredded mozzarella cheese to the bowl. Season with salt and pepper to taste. Mix well to combine.

8. Spoon the spinach and cheese mixture into the hollowed-out zucchini halves, pressing down gently to pack it in.

9. Place the stuffed zucchini halves in the prepared baking dish.

10. Bake in the preheated oven for 20-25 minutes, or until the zucchini is tender and the cheese is melted and bubbly. Remove from the oven and let the stuffed zucchini cool for a few minutes before serving. Garnish with chopped fresh basil leaves if desired.

87. Baked eggplant with tomato sauce and cheese

Ingredients:
- 2 medium-sized eggplants
- 2 tablespoons olive oil
- Salt and pepper to taste
- 1 cup marinara sauce or tomato sauce
- 1 cup shredded mozzarella cheese
- 1/4 cup grated Parmesan cheese
- Fresh basil leaves, chopped, for garnish (optional)

Instructions:
1. Preheat your oven to 400°F (200°C). Grease a baking dish with olive oil or cooking spray.

2. Wash the eggplants and slice them into rounds, about 1/4 to 1/2 inch thick.

3. Place the eggplant slices on a baking sheet lined with parchment paper. Brush both sides of the eggplant slices with olive oil and season with salt and pepper.

4. Bake the eggplant slices in the preheated oven for 15-20 minutes, flipping halfway through, until they are tender and lightly golden brown.

5. Remove the eggplant slices from the oven and reduce the oven temperature to 350°F (175°C).

6. In the prepared baking dish, spread a thin layer of marinara sauce or tomato sauce on the bottom.

7. Arrange half of the baked eggplant slices in a single layer over the sauce.

8. Spoon more marinara sauce or tomato sauce over the eggplant slices, then sprinkle half of the shredded mozzarella cheese and half of the grated Parmesan cheese on top.

9. Repeat with the remaining eggplant slices, sauce, and cheese.

10. Bake in the preheated oven for 20-25 minutes, or until the cheese is melted and bubbly.

11. Remove from the oven and let the baked eggplant cool for a few minutes before serving. Garnish with chopped fresh basil leaves if desired.

Enjoy your delicious baked eggplant with tomato sauce and cheese as a flavorful and comforting dish!

88. Vegetarian pho

Ingredients:
For the broth:
- 8 cups vegetable broth
- 1 onion, halved
- 1-inch piece of ginger, sliced
- 2 star anise
- 2 cinnamon sticks
- 4 cloves
- 2 cardamom pods
- 1 teaspoon coriander seeds
- 1 teaspoon fennel seeds
- 1 tablespoon soy sauce or tamari
- 1 tablespoon maple syrup or brown sugar
- Salt to taste

For the pho:
- 8 oz (225g) rice noodles
- 1 cup sliced shiitake mushrooms
- 1 cup sliced tofu or seitan
- 2 cups bean sprouts
- 1 cup sliced bok choy or baby spinach
- 1/2 cup thinly sliced onion
- 1/4 cup chopped fresh cilantro
- 1/4 cup chopped fresh mint
- 1/4 cup chopped fresh basil
- Lime wedges, for serving
- Sriracha or chili sauce, for serving (optional)
- Hoisin sauce, for serving (optional)

Instructions:

1. In a large pot, combine the vegetable broth, halved onion, sliced ginger, star anise, cinnamon sticks, cloves, cardamom pods, coriander seeds, and fennel seeds. Bring to a boil, then reduce the heat to low and simmer for 30 minutes to 1 hour to infuse the flavors.

2. Strain the broth through a fine-mesh sieve into another pot. Discard the solids. Return the strained broth to the stove and keep warm over low heat. Stir in the soy sauce or tamari, maple syrup or brown sugar, and salt to taste.

3. Meanwhile, cook the rice noodles according to the package instructions. Drain and rinse with cold water.

4. Divide the cooked rice noodles among serving bowls. Top with sliced shiitake mushrooms, sliced tofu or seitan, bean sprouts, sliced bok choy or baby spinach, and thinly sliced onion.

5. Ladle the hot broth over the noodles and vegetables in each bowl.

6. Serve the vegetarian pho hot, garnished with chopped fresh cilantro, mint, and basil. Serve with lime wedges, sriracha or chili sauce, and hoisin sauce on the side, if desired.

Enjoy your flavorful and comforting vegetarian pho!

89. Tofu lettuce wraps with peanut sauce

Ingredients:
- 1 block extra-firm tofu, pressed and cubed
- 2 tbsp sesame oil
- 2 cloves garlic, minced
- 1 inch ginger, grated
- 1 red bell pepper, thinly sliced
- 1 cup shredded carrots
- 1 cup bean sprouts
- 8-10 large lettuce leaves (such as romaine or bibb)

Peanut Sauce:
- 1/4 cup creamy peanut butter
- 2 tbsp low-sodium soy sauce
- 2 tbsp rice vinegar
- 1 tbsp honey
- 1 tsp sesame oil
- 1 tsp grated ginger
- 1-2 tbsp water to thin

Instructions:
1. Make the peanut sauce by whisking together all the sauce ingredients until smooth. Add water as needed to reach desired consistency. Set aside.

2. In a large skillet or wok, heat the sesame oil over medium-high heat. Add the tofu cubes and cook for 5-7 minutes, turning occasionally, until lightly browned on all sides.

3. Add the garlic and ginger to the pan and cook for 1 minute until fragrant.

4. Stir in the bell pepper, carrots and bean sprouts. Cook for 2-3 minutes until vegetables are tender-crisp.

5. To serve, place a few spoonfuls of the tofu and vegetable mixture into a lettuce leaf. Drizzle with the peanut sauce.

6. Wrap the lettuce around the filling and enjoy!

90. Lentil and vegetable stuffed peppers

Ingredients:
- 6 bell peppers, halved lengthwise and seeds removed
- 1 cup dry brown or green lentils, rinsed
- 2 cups vegetable broth
- 1 tbsp olive oil
- 1 onion, diced
- 3 cloves garlic, minced
- 1 cup diced zucchini
- 1 cup diced mushrooms
- 1 tsp dried oregano
- 1 tsp dried basil
- 1/2 tsp smoked paprika
- Salt and pepper to taste
- 1/2 cup shredded mozzarella cheese (optional)

Instructions:

1. Preheat oven to 375°F. Place the pepper halves cut-side up in a baking dish and set aside.

2. In a medium saucepan, combine the lentils and vegetable broth. Bring to a boil, then reduce heat and simmer for 15-20 minutes until lentils are tender. Drain any excess liquid.

3. In a skillet, heat the olive oil over medium heat. Add the onion and sauté for 3-4 minutes until translucent.

4. Add the garlic, zucchini, and mushrooms. Cook for 5-7 minutes, stirring occasionally, until vegetables are tender.

5. Stir the cooked lentils into the vegetable mixture. Add the oregano, basil, smoked paprika, salt and pepper. Mix well.

6. Spoon the lentil-vegetable filling into the pepper halves, packing it in tightly.

7. If using, sprinkle the shredded mozzarella over the top of the stuffed peppers.

8. Bake for 25-30 minutes, until the peppers are tender.

9. Serve hot. Enjoy!

91. Stuffed squash with wild rice and cranberries

Ingredients:
- 2 acorn squash, halved and seeds removed
- 1 cup wild rice, rinsed
- 2 cups vegetable or chicken broth
- 1 tbsp olive oil
- 1 onion, diced
- 2 cloves garlic, minced
- 1 cup diced celery
- 1 cup diced mushrooms
- 1/2 cup dried cranberries
- 1/4 cup chopped pecans
- 1 tsp dried thyme
- Salt and pepper to taste
- 1/4 cup crumbled feta cheese (optional)

Instructions:
1. Preheat oven to 400°F. Place the squash halves cut-side up on a baking sheet. Bake for 30-40 minutes, until tender when pierced with a fork.

2. In a medium saucepan, combine the wild rice and broth. Bring to a boil, then reduce heat and simmer for 30-35 minutes, until rice is tender. Drain any excess liquid.

3. In a skillet, heat the olive oil over medium heat. Add the onion and sauté for 3-4 minutes until translucent.

4. Add the garlic, celery, and mushrooms. Cook for 5-7 minutes, stirring occasionally, until vegetables are tender.

5. Stir the cooked wild rice into the vegetable mixture. Add the cranberries, pecans, and thyme. Season with salt and pepper.

6. Scoop the wild rice stuffing into the baked squash halves, packing it in tightly.

7. If using, sprinkle the crumbled feta cheese over the top of the stuffed squash.

8. Return the stuffed squash to the oven and bake for an additional 10-15 minutes, until heated through.

9. Serve hot. Enjoy!

92. Vegetable and tofu curry

Ingredients:
- 1 block extra-firm tofu, pressed and cubed
- 2 tbsp coconut oil
- 1 onion, diced
- 3 cloves garlic, minced
- 1 tbsp grated fresh ginger
- 2 tsp curry powder
- 1 tsp ground cumin
- 1 tsp ground coriander
- 1/2 tsp ground turmeric
- 1/4 tsp cayenne pepper (or to taste)
- 1 cup diced carrots
- 1 cup diced cauliflower florets
- 1 cup diced potatoes
- 1 cup diced bell pepper
- 1 (13.5 oz) can coconut milk
- 1 cup vegetable broth
- 1 tsp salt
- 1/4 cup chopped fresh cilantro
- Cooked basmati rice, for serving

Instructions:

1. In a large skillet or wok, heat the coconut oil over medium-high heat. Add the cubed tofu and cook for 5-7 minutes, turning occasionally, until lightly browned on all sides. Transfer tofu to a plate.

2. In the same pan, add the onion and sauté for 3-4 minutes until translucent.

3. Add the garlic and ginger and cook for 1 minute until fragrant.

4. Stir in the curry powder, cumin, coriander, turmeric, and cayenne. Cook for 1 minute to toast the spices.

5. Add the carrots, cauliflower, potatoes, and bell pepper. Sauté for 5-7 minutes until vegetables start to soften.

6. Pour in the coconut milk and vegetable broth. Bring to a simmer and cook for 10-15 minutes, until vegetables are tender.

7. Gently stir the cooked tofu back into the curry. Season with salt. Remove from heat and stir in the chopped cilantro. Serve the vegetable and tofu curry over steamed basmati rice.

93. Spinach and feta stuffed mushrooms

Ingredients:
- 16-20 medium cremini or button mushrooms, stems removed and finely chopped
- 2 tbsp olive oil
- 1/2 onion, finely diced
- 2 cloves garlic, minced
- 2 cups fresh spinach, chopped
- 4 oz crumbled feta cheese
- 2 tbsp breadcrumbs
- 1 tbsp lemon juice
- 1/4 tsp dried oregano
- Salt and pepper to taste

Instructions:

1. Preheat oven to 375°F. Clean the mushrooms and remove the stems, finely chopping the stems.

2. In a skillet, heat the olive oil over medium heat. Add the chopped mushroom stems, onion, and garlic. Sauté for 3-4 minutes until softened.

3. Add the chopped spinach and cook for 2-3 minutes until wilted. Remove from heat and let cool slightly.

4. In a medium bowl, combine the sautéed mushroom stem mixture, feta cheese, breadcrumbs, lemon juice, and oregano. Season with salt and pepper.

5. Stuff the mushroom caps evenly with the spinach and feta filling, packing it in tightly.

6. Arrange the stuffed mushrooms on a baking sheet.

7. Bake for 12-15 minutes, until the mushrooms are tender and the filling is hot.

8. Serve the spinach and feta stuffed mushrooms warm. Enjoy!

Tips:
- You can use a small spoon or your fingers to stuff the mushroom caps.
- For extra flavor, you can add a sprinkle of grated Parmesan cheese on top before baking.
- These make a great appetizer or side dish.

94. Quinoa stuffed tomatoes

Ingredients:
- 6 medium tomatoes
- 1 cup cooked quinoa
- 1/2 cup crumbled feta cheese
- 1/4 cup chopped fresh basil
- 2 tbsp olive oil
- 2 cloves garlic, minced
- 1/4 tsp red pepper flakes (optional)
- Salt and pepper to taste

Instructions:

1. Preheat oven to 375°F.

2. Slice the tops off the tomatoes and scoop out the insides, leaving a 1/4-inch shell. Finely chop the scooped out tomato flesh.

3. In a medium bowl, combine the chopped tomato flesh, cooked quinoa, feta cheese, basil, olive oil, garlic, and red pepper flakes (if using). Season with salt and pepper.

4. Stuff the quinoa mixture evenly into the tomato shells, packing it in tightly.

5. Arrange the stuffed tomatoes in a baking dish.

6. Bake for 20-25 minutes, until the tomatoes are softened and the filling is hot.

7. Serve the quinoa stuffed tomatoes warm. Enjoy!

Tips:
- For extra flavor, you can add other chopped veggies like onion, bell pepper, or spinach to the quinoa filling.
- Top the stuffed tomatoes with a sprinkle of Parmesan cheese before baking.
- These make a great vegetarian main dish or side.

95. Vegetable pad see ew

Ingredients:
- 8 oz wide rice noodles
- 2 tbsp soy sauce
- 1 tbsp oyster sauce
- 1 tbsp brown sugar
- 1 tsp sesame oil
- 2 tbsp vegetable oil
- 3 cloves garlic, minced
- 1 cup broccoli florets
- 1 cup sliced mushrooms
- 1 cup shredded carrots
- 2 cups chopped Chinese broccoli or kale
- 2 eggs, lightly beaten
- 1 tbsp soy sauce, for serving
- Chopped cilantro, for garnish

Instructions:
1. Soak the rice noodles in hot water for 15-20 minutes until softened. Drain and set aside.

2. In a small bowl, whisk together the 2 tbsp soy sauce, oyster sauce, brown sugar, and sesame oil. Set aside.

3. Heat the vegetable oil in a large wok or skillet over high heat. Add the garlic and stir-fry for 30 seconds until fragrant.

4. Add the broccoli, mushrooms, and carrots. Stir-fry for 2-3 minutes until vegetables start to soften.

5. Push the vegetables to the side of the wok and pour the beaten eggs into the center. Let cook for 1 minute, then scramble the eggs.

6. Add the softened rice noodles and the sauce mixture. Toss everything together, stirring constantly, for 2-3 minutes until the noodles are evenly coated and heated through.

7. Stir in the Chinese broccoli or kale and cook for 1-2 minutes more until the greens are wilted.

8. Remove from heat and serve the vegetable pad see ew immediately, with extra soy sauce on the side. Garnish with chopped cilantro.

96. Tofu and vegetable kebabs with peanut sauce

Ingredients:
Kebabs:
- 1 block extra-firm tofu, pressed and cut into 1-inch cubes
- 1 red bell pepper, cut into 1-inch pieces
- 1 zucchini, cut into 1-inch pieces
- 1 red onion, cut into 1-inch pieces
- 8 oz mushrooms, halved
- Wooden or metal skewers

Peanut Sauce:
- 1/4 cup creamy peanut butter
- 2 tbsp low-sodium soy sauce
- 2 tbsp rice vinegar
- 1 tbsp honey
- 1 tsp sesame oil
- 1 tsp grated ginger
- 2-3 tbsp water, to thin

Instructions:
1. Make the peanut sauce by whisking together all the sauce ingredients until smooth. Add water as needed to reach desired consistency. Set aside.

2. Preheat grill or grill pan to medium-high heat.

3. Thread the tofu, bell pepper, zucchini, onion, and mushrooms onto the skewers, alternating the ingredients.

4. Grill the kebabs for 10-12 minutes, turning occasionally, until the vegetables are tender and the tofu is lightly charred.

5. Serve the grilled tofu and vegetable kebabs immediately, with the peanut sauce drizzled over the top or served on the side for dipping.

Tips:
- Soak wooden skewers in water for 30 minutes before using to prevent burning.
- You can use any combination of vegetables you like, such as eggplant, cherry tomatoes, or pineapple.
- For extra flavor, marinate the tofu in a bit of soy sauce, garlic, and ginger before threading onto the skewers.

97. Stuffed sweet potatoes with black beans and corn

Ingredients:
- 4 medium sweet potatoes
- 1 (15 oz) can black beans, drained and rinsed
- 1 cup frozen corn kernels
- 1/2 cup salsa
- 1 tsp chili powder
- 1/2 tsp ground cumin
- 1/4 tsp garlic powder
- Salt and pepper to taste
- 1/2 cup shredded cheddar or monterey jack cheese (optional)
- Chopped cilantro for garnish

Instructions:

1. Preheat oven to 400°F. Pierce the sweet potatoes several times with a fork and place on a baking sheet. Bake for 45-60 minutes, until very soft when squeezed.

2. Remove the sweet potatoes from the oven and let cool slightly. Cut each potato in half lengthwise.

3. Scoop the flesh out of the sweet potato halves, leaving about 1/4 inch of flesh attached to the skin to create a "boat".

4. In a medium bowl, mash the scooped sweet potato flesh. Stir in the black beans, corn, salsa, chili powder, cumin, garlic powder, and salt and pepper to taste.

5. Spoon the black bean and sweet potato mixture back into the sweet potato skins, packing it in tightly.

6. If using, sprinkle the shredded cheese over the top of the stuffed sweet potatoes.

7. Return the stuffed sweet potatoes to the oven and bake for an additional 10-15 minutes, until heated through and cheese is melted.

8. Serve the stuffed sweet potatoes warm, garnished with chopped cilantro.

Enjoy this easy and nutritious vegetarian stuffed sweet potato dish!

98. Vegetarian sushi rolls with avocado and cucumber

Ingredients:
- 1 cup short-grain sushi rice
- 2 tbsp rice vinegar
- 1 tsp sugar
- 1/2 tsp salt
- 4 sheets nori (seaweed sheets)
- 1 avocado, sliced
- 1 cucumber, peeled and cut into thin strips
- 1/4 cup toasted sesame seeds

Dipping Sauce:
- 2 tbsp low-sodium soy sauce
- 1 tbsp rice vinegar
- 1 tsp sesame oil
- 1 tsp grated ginger

Instructions:

1. Cook the sushi rice according to package instructions. Transfer to a large bowl and stir in the rice vinegar, sugar, and salt. Let cool completely.

2. Place a sheet of nori on a bamboo sushi mat or clean surface. Spread about 1/2 cup of the cooled sushi rice evenly over the nori, leaving a 1-inch border at the top.

3. Arrange a few slices of avocado and cucumber strips in a line across the center of the rice.

4. Starting from the bottom, tightly roll up the nori around the fillings, using the bamboo mat to help you roll it up. Moisten the top edge with a bit of water to seal the roll.

5. Repeat with the remaining nori sheets and fillings.

6. Slice each sushi roll into 6-8 pieces using a sharp knife. Wet the knife between cuts to prevent sticking.

7. For the dipping sauce, whisk together all the sauce ingredients in a small bowl.

8. Arrange the sushi rolls on a plate and sprinkle with the toasted sesame seeds. Serve immediately with the dipping sauce on the side.

Enjoy these fresh and flavorful vegetarian sushi rolls!

99. Tofu and vegetable bibimbap bowl

Ingredients:
- 1 block extra-firm tofu, pressed and cubed
- 2 tbsp sesame oil, divided
- 2 cups cooked brown rice
- 1 cup shredded carrots
- 1 cup thinly sliced mushrooms
- 1 cup baby spinach
- 1 cup bean sprouts
- 2 scallions, thinly sliced
- 2 eggs (optional)
- Gochujang or sriracha, for serving

Bibimbap Sauce:
- 2 tbsp gochujang (Korean chili paste)
- 1 tbsp soy sauce
- 1 tbsp rice vinegar
- 1 tsp sesame oil
- 1 tsp honey
- 1 tsp grated ginger

Instructions:

1. In a large skillet, heat 1 tbsp sesame oil over medium-high heat. Add the tofu cubes and cook for 5-7 minutes, turning occasionally, until lightly browned on all sides. Transfer to a plate.

2. In the same skillet, heat the remaining 1 tbsp sesame oil. Add the carrots, mushrooms, spinach, and bean sprouts. Sauté for 3-4 minutes until vegetables are tender-crisp.

3. Make the bibimbap sauce by whisking together all the sauce ingredients in a small bowl.

4. To assemble the bowls, divide the cooked brown rice among 4 serving bowls. Top each with the sautéed vegetables, tofu, and scallions.

5. If desired, fry or soft-boil 2 eggs and place one on top of each bibimbap bowl. Drizzle the bibimbap sauce over the top of each bowl. Serve the tofu and vegetable bibimbap immediately, with extra gochujang or sriracha on the side.

Stir everything together before eating to combine all the flavors. Enjoy this colorful and nutritious Korean-inspired vegetarian dish!

100. Lentil and vegetable biryani

Ingredients:
- 1 cup brown or green lentils, rinsed
- 2 cups vegetable broth
- 2 tbsp olive oil
- 1 onion, diced
- 3 cloves garlic, minced
- 1 tbsp grated fresh ginger
- 2 tsp garam masala
- 1 tsp ground cumin
- 1 tsp ground coriander
- 1/2 tsp turmeric
- 1/4 tsp cayenne pepper (or to taste)
- 1 cup diced cauliflower
- 1 cup diced sweet potato
- 1 cup frozen peas
- 1 cup basmati rice
- 1/4 cup chopped cilantro
- Juice of 1 lemon
- Salt and pepper to taste

Instructions:
1. In a medium saucepan, combine the lentils and vegetable broth. Bring to a boil, then reduce heat and simmer for 15-20 minutes until lentils are tender. Drain any excess liquid.

2. In a large skillet or pot, heat the olive oil over medium heat. Add the onion and sauté for 3-4 minutes until translucent.

3. Stir in the garlic, ginger, garam masala, cumin, coriander, turmeric, and cayenne. Cook for 1 minute until fragrant.

4. Add the cauliflower, sweet potato, and peas. Sauté for 5-7 minutes until vegetables are tender-crisp.

5. Stir the cooked lentils into the vegetable mixture. Season with salt and pepper.

6. In a separate pot, cook the basmati rice according to package instructions.

7. To serve, place a portion of the lentil and vegetable biryani in a bowl. Top with a scoop of the cooked basmati rice. Garnish with chopped cilantro and a squeeze of lemon juice.

*As you come to the end of **"100 Vegetarian Recipes for Soothing Diverticulitis Symptoms,"** we hope you feel empowered and inspired to take control of your health through delicious, plant-based meals. Throughout this journey, we've explored the intersection of vegetarian cuisine and digestive wellness, offering a diverse array of recipes designed to support individuals living with diverticulitis.*

Managing diverticulitis can present challenges, but by prioritizing gentle, gut-friendly ingredients, we can alleviate symptoms, promote healing, and enhance overall well-being. Whether you've been following a vegetarian lifestyle for years or are just beginning to explore plant-based eating, we hope you've discovered new favorites and gained valuable insights into nourishing your body with compassion and intention.

As you continue on your journey, remember that food is not only sustenance but also a source of joy, connection, and healing. Experiment with flavors, embrace seasonal ingredients, and listen to your body's unique needs as you craft meals that nourish both body and soul.

We extend our heartfelt gratitude to you for choosing this cookbook as a companion on your path to wellness. May these recipes bring warmth to your kitchen, comfort to your belly, and vitality to your life. Here's to vibrant health, delicious food, and thriving with diverticulitis. Bon appétit!